Semantic-Pragmatic
LANGUAGE DISORDER

Charlotte Firth

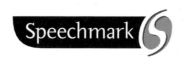

Telford Road • Bicester • Oxon OX26 4LQ • UK

Editor's Note

For the sake of clarity alone, in this pack we have used 'he' to refer to the child.

Published by
Speechmark Publishing Ltd, Telford Road, Bicester, Oxon OX26 4LQ
United Kingdom
www.speechmark.net

© Charlotte Firth & Katherine Venkatesh, 1999
First published 1999
Reprinted 2001, 2002, 2003

002-3342/Printed in the United Kingdom/1030
British Library Cataloguing in Publication Data
Firth, Charlotte,
    Introductory manual
    Part 1 Charlotte Firth, Katherine Venkatesh
    1. Speech disorders in children 2. Speech disorders in children – Diagnosis
    3. Speech therapy for children
    I. Title II. Venkatesh, Katherine
    616.9'2855'06

ISBN for Part 1: 0 86388 326 5
ISBN for complete set of 3 volumes: ISBN 0 86388 329 X
ISBN for Part 2: 0 86388 327 3
ISBN for Part 3: 0 86388 328 1
*Previously published by Winslow Press Ltd under ISBN 0 86388 240 4 (Part 1),
0 86388 241 2 (Part 2), 0 86388 242 0 (Part 3), 0 86388 203 X (complete set)*

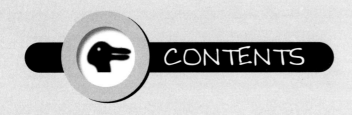

CONTENTS

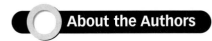
About the Authors

Charlotte Firth qualified as a speech & language therapist in 1989 from Leeds Metropolitan University. She has always worked in Yorkshire, initially with adults and children in clinic and hospital settings, but she began to specialize in paediatric work in 1990. In May 1990, she became a part-time research assistant at Leeds Metropolitan University, working with Dr Michael Perkins on a pilot study to investigate 'the use and comprehension of modal auxiliary verbs in children with a Semantic–Pragmatic language disorder'. In 1992, after another year working with children in schools and clinics, she took up her present post in Scarborough. She now works predominantly with special needs children in mainstream schools

Katherine Venkatesh (née Southwell) qualified as a speech & language therapist in 1986 from Leeds Metropolitan University. Since then, she has worked in North Derbyshire and Scarborough, specializing in working with children in a variety of settings. She has also qualified as a course tutor for the Derbyshire Language Scheme. Her involvement with this project arose from a chance remark in Summer 1996, when she offered to provide some pictures for her colleague Charlotte Firth's therapy programmes. At present, she is not working as a speech & language therapist as she is a full-time mother.

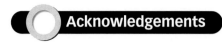 **Acknowledgements**

Firstly, we would like to acknowledge the help given by those who reviewed the first draft of the whole pack, Helen Harron, Mary Jones, Valerie Kingston and Mick Perkins.

Our thanks go also to our partners, Matt and Ashok, for all their support.

Charlotte would particularly like to thank John Lea for all his time, patience and technical expertise in producing the initial pack. She would also like to thank Mick Perkins for introducing her to the world of 'Semantic–Pragmatic' disorder.

In addition, Kathy would like to thank Rosemary Blakesley for the help and support she has always given.

Finally, thanks to the children and families who have provided us with the inspiration needed to produce this pack.

Charlotte Firth and **Kathy Venkatesh**

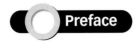 **Preface**

Semantic–Pragmatic Disorder: my first encounter with this term was as a student, just before my final exams. It was suggested that a question about the disorder would be likely to appear in our final year Speech Pathology examination. Following a hasty trawl through papers circulating at the time, I was relieved to find a question that summer (1989) which read: 'What might be the most relevant approach to intervention with a boy of ten with a Semantic–Pragmatic disorder?' I attempted to answer that particular question (I would enjoy reading my response now!) and my interest in the disorder was born.

Soon after qualifying, I worked as a research assistant at Leeds Metropolitan University on a project investigating how children with a Semantic–Pragmatic disorder understood and used modal auxiliary verbs. My knowledge and thoughts regarding the disorder started to develop and I began work that was later to form the basis for this resource pack. By summer 1996, I had developed the initial pack and Kathy joined me in the project. We redesigned the therapy ideas and adapted them to include Kathy's illustrations and handouts.

Today there is a great deal of published material regarding this language disorder. However, those in day-to-day contact with the children often seem frustrated by the lack of a simple framework to help identify, treat and manage this type of difficulty. I hope this resource pack will help meet this need to some degree. It does not purport to cover the wide range of theoretical models and therapy approaches that can be employed when working with individuals who have this type of disability. Most of the information in the pack has been acquired through time spent with these children and their families. The therapy ideas are merely a selection of the activities that have proved useful when working with children of this type.

Charlotte Firth
Malton, 1998

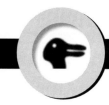

INTRODUCTION

A discussion regarding the disorder

Section 1

INTRODUCTION

There have been many papers, articles, reports and discussions in relation to Semantic–Pragmatic Disorder, and the subject still creates a great deal of interest. The following points summarize certain issues that recur concerning this disorder. Readers who anticipate some difficulty with the terminology used in this Introduction are advised to read first *Section 2 (Questions & Answers)*, which will answer a number of the most frequently asked questions.

Interest in the UK in this 'new' disorder developed in the early 1980s. Several papers (including Culloden *et al*, 1986; Jones *et al*, 1986) were presented at the Invalid Children's Aid Nationwide Conference in 1986. These papers attempted to describe what did and did not constitute a disorder of this type. They also detailed how semantic, pragmatic (and syntactic) skills were affected in this type of language difficulty.

It soon became clear that it was not sufficient to detail characteristic features of this disorder, as the profile of the disorder changed over time. A characteristic pattern of semantic and pragmatic impairments became apparent. Initially, the child would be late to start speaking and would then use a great deal of echolalic language, often without comprehension. Later, the child would use relatively well formed language, the echoing would diminish but there would still be difficulties with comprehension. By around seven years of age, the child would understand more but have difficulties with social interaction (Shields *et al*, 1996). The child would speak inappropriately (Bishop & Adams, 1989), frequently change the topic and have difficulties maintaining a normal conversation (Adams & Bishop, 1989). When older, the child would have difficulties understanding the rules of social situations and conversations and interpret language very literally (Bishop & Adams, 1992, Kerbel *et al*, 1996). He would have continuing difficulties comprehending non-literal language, such as idioms: for example, "She flew across the room" (Kerbel & Grunwell, 1998).

◯ Semantic–Pragmatic Disorder: Origins

Those who work with language-disordered children seek to classify linguistic problems, possibly in an attempt to plan therapy using informed judgements. Boucher (1998) feels that the use of Semantic–Pragmatic Disorder as a diagnostic category exists partly so that therapists can describe the child's difficulties and also to 'point the therapist towards goals and methods of intervention'.

Descriptive terms and labels change over time as ideas are refined and in the light of theoretical knowledge. There seemed to have been descriptions of what were semantic–pragmatic disorder-type difficulties without actually using this label. For instance, a paper entitled 'Language Without Communication: a Case Study', Blank *et al* (1979) described John (3 years 3 months). He did not interact with anyone other than his parents, but was age-appropriate in non-verbal areas.

He started to speak late, did not enjoy games such as 'peek-a-boo' and had sing-song prosody. His speech was clear and grammatically well formed.

Cromer (1981) felt that there was a need to identify difficulties in many areas, including cognition, phonology, syntax, *semantics* and *pragmatics*. This would then lead to a fuller understanding of language disorders. Rapin and Allen (1983) were also frustrated by the lack of means available to classify child language disabilities. They attempted to group these children into seven different syndrome types, one of which they named Semantic–Pragmatic Syndrome Without Autism. The development of this label was to start what has amounted to 15 years of discussion, debate and research into this type of language disorder. Rapin and Allen noted that these children produced syntactically well formed speech with good phonology, but had difficulty following conversations and had a striking inability to engage in communicative discourse.

Semantic–Pragmatic Disorder, Asperger Syndrome and Autism: How do they Differ?

This question has generated a great deal of research and (often heated) debate. Many argue that a child with Semantic–Pragmatic Disorder has a degree of autism and should not be identified as being apart or different from those with Asperger Syndrome or classic autism. Bishop (1989) attempted to describe autism, Asperger Syndrome and Semantic–Pragmatic Disorder as discrete disorders but with overlapping characteristics. A child with autism *is* likely to present with the typical characteristics of a Semantic–Pragmatic Disorder. Kanner (1943) recognized that disordered language was a cardinal symptom of infantile autism. He described autistic language as characterized by echolalia, metaphorical substitutions, transfers of meaning through analogy and generalization, literalness, pronoun reversals and verbal negations (Kanner, 1946). This is a familiar description.

Wing (1988) identified a triad of impairments in autism. She described a spectrum of deficits along three continuums of social functioning. The first of these was with social *recognition*, 'the ability to recognise that people are the most interesting and potentially rewarding features of the environment'. She felt that, at the milder end of the continuum, this was best described 'as a poverty of the grasp of the subtle rules of interaction and a lack of perceptiveness towards others'. Secondly, she described varying levels of difficulty with social *imagination and understanding*. This deficit inhibits the ability to understand the meaning and purpose of the actions of others, as it 'affects the ability to recognise what others may know or feel'. Thirdly, she detailed deficits in social *communication*, again at a milder level, this would impair 'the ability to recognise the needs of conversational partners'. Clearly, many children described as having a Semantic–Pragmatic disorder do exhibit these features to some degree.

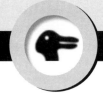

INTRODUCTION

Perhaps a different diagnostic category evolved as children with milder difficulties did not fully satisfy the criteria for typical autism. Brook and Bowler (1992) felt, however, that focusing attention on the communication impairments and labelling them 'semantic–pragmatic' did not fully address these children's problems as any underlying degree of autism was then ignored. They felt that this may have happened when, for example, the child used eye contact or displayed prosocial behaviours. Autism was then disregarded whereas, if these features had been recognized as present but *inappropriate*, a more accurate diagnosis would have been made.

Boucher (1998) felt that, if we are to decide whether Semantic–Pragmatic Disorder is a valid diagnostic category, we should look closely at the way we describe both autism and specific language impairment. It may be possible then to decide whether it falls in, or perhaps between, the two categories. Boucher first described both autism and specific language impairment in terms of a 'syndrome' ('a unitary disorder [in which] diverse signs and symptoms stem from a single cause'). She stressed that semantic–pragmatic disorder could not form part of the autistic diagnostic category under this description as it would then be classified as 'mild autism'. This diagnosis would then be redundant as Asperger Syndrome is already used to describe mild autism. Nor could it be classified under specific language impairment if this is described as a syndrome, as we do not usually describe language disorders in this way since we know from our experience of acquired disorders that they do not have a unitary cause.

Boucher then went on to describe autism and SPD (Semantic–Pragmatic Disorder) within a 'spectrum of subtypes' concept. She noted that '… for SPD to be established as a distinct subtype of autism, clear and reliable differences as well as similarities would have to be established within the typical behavioural profiles of children with SPD as opposed to children with Asperger disorder kanner-type autism" (and other 'pervasive developmental disorders'). Semantic–Pragmatic Disorder could be a subtype of this type, and this is how Bishop (1989, mentioned above) tried to analyse the disorder.

Finally, Boucher described autism and Semantic–Pragmatic Disorder using the concept of a 'continuum of impairment'. She felt this idea was useful as it could then identify degrees of impairment in a range of developmental areas and individual profiles could be established. Equally, however, any specific diagnosis would be hard to establish using this model as there is scope for an almost endless range of variations. Autism and Semantic–Pragmatic Disorder would both then become nonentities (although we know that certain characteristics tend to group together). Boucher's final prediction was that Semantic–Pragmatic Disorder will prove to be a subtype of autism.

Perhaps if we look to the causes of what we will call 'autistic spectrum disorders' this may help with diagnosis.

Autistic Spectrum Disorders: Shared Deficits

If we consider what may cause the shared social and pragmatic impairments, this may reveal a common basis for these disorders. It appears that the majority of people with autistic spectrum disorders have some degree of difficulty processing sensory input, and what they see, hear, touch, smell and taste is not dealt with in the usual way. Information, for instance a sound, is received, but it is perceived in an unusual way. Boucher (1998) hypothesized that, 'SPD shares with both Asperger disorder and Kanner-type autism a specific deficit in information processing which impairs the registration and organization of complex experience, and to generate behaviour and to plan'.

We make sense of our world by analysing our experiences. We can deduce, infer and hypothesize by using, for instance, our judgement of the situations we are in, the people present and our knowledge of experiences we have already had. It is this ability, to draw information together at a 'central' level, that is impaired in autistic spectrum disorders. This skill usually starts to develop from birth and everyone differs in their level and type of 'central processing' ability. When there are significant deficits in this area, however, this can disrupt normal development. Frith (1989) stressed that, 'Just this particular fault in the mechanics of the mind can explain the essential features of Autism. The rest is secondary.'

Any characteristic feature of autism can be explained using this model. Examples might be the need for routine (necessary if it is difficult or even impossible to make sense of new information), restricted diets (again the threat of the unknown) or fear of new people (if it is hard to interpret their thoughts or how they might act).

How, then, does this difficulty in 'organising, drawing together information to make it coherent and meaningful' (Frith, 1989), affect someone's language skills?

Central Processing Skills and Linguistic Development

Semantic Skills

Semantics is the study of meaning in language (Crystal, 1985). A child develops his ability to attach meanings to words by gradually refining his concepts about his environment and the things he experiences. Early words are overgeneralized; for instance, initially 'male' may equal 'daddy' only, and then this term is applied for a short while to any man the child sees. As the child experiences more and develops concepts about the world, an increasingly complex vocabulary develops. If the child cannot draw information together to devise new ideas in this way, semantic development is unusual.

When a child has a central processing disorder there is a need for familiarity, resulting in a tendency for the child to develop first words that relate to his interests and personal needs. However, these words may not be very useful in a communicative sense. The child may, for instance, enjoy reciting words, for his own pleasure. There is less need to develop words such as 'mummy' if people are not a very important feature of the child's environment.

He may also remember words without having a true understanding of them. Jarrold *et al* (1997) studied a sample of 120 children with autistic spectrum disorders. They found that 'Children's scores on the WFT [a word finding test] were significantly higher than their scores on the BPVS [a test of receptive vocabulary].' Children with a Semantic–Pragmatic Disorder may learn many words in relation to particular areas, accumulated using their often excellent ability to memorize information. Paul (1987) mentions that 'Autistic children often develop large vocabularies and some take an obsessive interest in words and word meanings.' This is in contrast to normal development, when the child builds up a vocabulary through developing and refining his knowledge of the world around him, this type of development being through, and in response to, his everyday, communicative needs.

Later in the child's life this method of accumulating a vocabulary has an effect on the way words are interpreted. If a word is acquired by rote rather than through a developing understanding of the world around him, the child may find it hard to accept how words vary in their meaning, depending on the other words in the phrase or the situation they are used in. It will also be hard for the child to accept additional non-literal meanings of words and phrases.

Difficulties interpreting people's thoughts and situations, may mean that, for example, 'nice', said in a sarcastic tone, will be misconstrued. Metaphor and other similar uses of language may also confuse the child as he cannot consider the wider picture and use situational factors, including the person's tone of voice and experiential knowledge to interpret the words at a less literal level. The child may interpret certain words in one particular way. For instance, he may be annoyed if someone tries to say that 'bay' is the colour of a horse, when he has previously found that it relates to the seaside, or that 'on' can relate to the vertical plane (for instance, a clock can be 'on' a wall) when he has been taught 'on' in the horizontal sense. The child's inability to be flexible in this way will mean he may find it hard to accept these multiple word meanings.

Language skills are gradually built up following certain rules; for instance, words relate to one another and are classified in certain ways. Grammatical development also has a rule-based system by which it develops. If the child has not generated language using these systems, but has tended rather to memorize whole or part phrases, his speech will actually be delayed echolalia. It will then be hard for him to retrieve individual words as they may be 'hidden' within a learnt phrase. Word-finding difficulties can then occur.

Pragmatic Skills

Pragmatics is the study of the way language is used, the choices made and the constraints encountered when language is used for social interaction (Crystal, 1985). Individuals who have difficulties drawing information together to make sense of the situations they are in are likely to have a pragmatic disorder. Other people will be confusing, and their actions potentially threatening, if it is difficult to construe what they may be thinking. This will be even more of a problem if the child finds it hard to process and understand speech. If he wants to converse, he will have little to guide him in his efforts. He may then use irrelevant language or dominate a conversation to feel more confident in his communicative attempts.

Non-verbal aspects of language, such as tone of voice and facial expression, will mean little to the child, as he will not have developed an understanding of these through experience. In short, this core inability to derive meaning by processing information at a central level can have anything from a mild to a devastating effect on pragmatic competence.

Syntactic Skills

Contrary to popular belief, it seems that children with a Semantic–Pragmatic Disorder do not always produce well formed, syntactically correct speech. As has been mentioned grammatical skills are normally built up and develop following a rule-based system. Children within the autistic spectrum tend to memorize language rather than develop it in this way. Where children described as having Semantic–Pragmatic Disorder seem to differ from those with autism and Asperger Syndrome is that there seems to be some correlation between the child's wish to be relevant and pertinent in conversation and the degree to which his speech becomes syntactically misformulated (although this seems to reach a peak at a certain age in these children). Consequently, those children with a lesser degree of the underlying deficit that causes the pragmatic disorder may produce phrases such as "The dog is barking to chase the cat" (a dog barking at a cat as he chases it) or "The maybe the if someone's inside the house and throw the key out outside, so might the man won't get in" (a man standing outside his house, who appears to have lost his keys).

This appears to be a result of the child struggling to produce a relevant response when he has only memorized whole phrases to help him do this. The child then tries to fit together segments or chunks of these phrases to formulate a good response (as he is partially aware of the needs of the listener and cares about their participation in the conversation to some degree). For instance, the following was produced as one continuous utterance: "They could be/a pool/ the boy's lying down/the girl's getting over/another pool" (a girl climbing out of a swimming pool oblivious to a boy in the pool who is shouting for help). The obliques in the quotation indicate where part phrases may have been used as the child attempted to get his message across.

In addition, the child may also exhibit 'false starts' as he tries to remember part and whole phrases; for instance: "After play, before play, I had it before, I had it before I had, I'll, I'll, see you after break."

Phonological Skills

Much has been made of the fact that children with a Semantic–Pragmatic Disorder do not have speech sound difficulties. If this is the case then it could be a result of the child memorizing speech he has heard, which, for the main part, is likely to be adult speech that is fully developed. Phonological skills usually follow a particular developmental route that is in step with all other areas of language development. Often children with Semantic–Pragmatic Disorder do not go through the usual developmental speech and language stages and this is given as a reason for the lack of normal phonological sound substitutions and/or disorders. However, processing difficulties can affect auditory skills and children may then internalize and copy speech as they have perceived it. The child may then produce rather unusual speech patterns, characterized by unusual, deviant phonological substitutions and structural abnormalities, such as producing only certain segments of words: for instance, "sman pa" (Postman Pat). Children may also produce very deviant phonological patterns and substitutions due to their processing disorder. These need to be appreciated as such and not necessarily as dyspraxic speech patterns (that is, expressive, motor programming difficulties).

◯ Semantic–Pragmatic Disorder, Asperger Syndrome and Autism: Should We Use Separate Labels?

The above labels and several others, such as High LEvel Language Disorder (HLLD) (Hockey, 1989) appear to detail almost the same characteristics. Central processing difficulties produce a range of impairments, including linguistic impairment, but it is too simplistic to say that these form a range from mild to moderate. This cognitive disorder can affect a range of developmental areas, each in a variety of ways to differing degrees (the continuum concept). For instance, a child may have affected visual skills as a consequence of having a heightened perception of patterns or colours and then have a mild degree of this difficulty. This facet of the child's functioning in combination with his levels ability and disability in other developmental areas, form the clinical picture for that child.

Gagnon *et al* (1997) argue that there is little point in creating a new category of disability when there is already a "well-defined diagnostic category (ie. high functioning autism) whose symptoms coincide with those of semantic–pragmatic syndrome …". However, classic or 'Kanner type' autistic disorder is diagnosed when a child has a certain set of characteristics each of which he exhibits to a specific degree. Confusion arises when a child has the same characteristics, but some or all of these typical features are exhibited to a milder degree. Such children then tend to have the most disordered areas of development labelled. Perhaps it is in response to this that a specific category (Semantic–Pragmatic Disorder) evolved, when evidently a certain subgroup of children had mostly linguistic deficits and less affected development in other areas.

We must not overlook, however, the fact that certain children can present with most of the features highlighted on a typical Semantic–Pragmatic checklist and not have the underlying cognitive deficits that also cause autism.

Cromer (1981) stresses: 'Some language-disordered individuals then, may be more profitably understood in terms of a deficit in the pragmatic component of their language system. This may be true of some autistic children as well as some children who do not share other features of autistic behaviour.' Rapin and Allen (1998) felt that some of the confusion in the differential diagnosis debate is a result of our tendency to classify at different levels of behaviour. The first and highest level is diagnostic, where 'autism' and 'specific language disorder' are both behavioural classifications. They stressed that language abilities form another, second level of classification and that, at this level, 'subtypes of the language deficits DLD [developmental language disorders] and autism/PDD [pervasive development disorder] overlap [and consequently] there is no justification for reifying SPD to the position of primary diagnosis'.

Certainly it appears that much of the confusion in 'labelling' arises from this point. It is quite nonsensical to debate whether two notions are the same or different if they describe separate levels of behaviour. We would be debating a similar point if we were trying to decide whether someone had tonsillitis *or a* sore throat. One is extremely likely to be a consequence of the other, but we must also be aware that it is possible at times to have a sore throat without it being due to tonsillitis.

A case in point would be a child with a specific word-finding difficulty. Such children often have severe pragmatic difficulties. For instance, they may say inappropriate things (as they cannot select words), join in conversations at the wrong time (as they start to speak when they have managed to think of what they need to say) and may deliver long monologues (as it may be easier to continue speaking once they have started). They may also develop rather repetitive interests and speech, as it will be easier to retrieve familiar words. They also clearly have semantic difficulties. This would demonstrate how a child could have the symptoms of a semantic and pragmatic disorder (the sore throat) without the underlying cause (the tonsillitis) being autism.

It is possible, however, that this group of children do not present with very early communicative problems, which the majority of children within the autistic spectrum exhibit. This does not mean, though, that it is incorrect to describe them as having semantic and pragmatic difficulties. Jarrold *et al* (1997) argue that autistic children's language deficits are cognitive rather than linguistic in origin. They note that, if they were linguistic, there would be phonological and articulatory difficulties present also, as these are 'almost always present in cases of specific language disorder'. However, as mentioned above, children with a central processing disorder can exhibit speech sound difficulties.

Firstly, these difficulties often present when the child has what appear to be specific difficulties processing the phonological components of speech. The child then makes imprecise copies of words and phrases he hears, becoming less precise the more he tries to memorize, so perhaps a single word may be relatively clear, but a rote learnt whole phrase or song will have many sound substitutions and 'muffled' pronunciations. Secondly, as the child often adopts a particular intonation pattern, for instance jerky syllable-timed speech, the sounds within the words may be articulated in an unusual way and speech will then sound odd at a phonetic level.

It seems therefore that it is almost impossible to differentiate children on the basis of the features of their particular developmental disorder. A possible solution could be to identify the *underlying cognitive deficit* and then use different labels to *describe* that child's particular difficulties. Then those that have mainly linguistic deficits would be labelled 'Semantic–Pragmatic', those with more significant social deficits but relatively intact language skills would be labelled 'Asperger Syndrome' and those with significantly affected skills in all areas of Wing's (1988) 'triad of impairments' could be said to have autism. Then a diagnosis of Semantic–Pragmatic Disorder would not exclude the underlying deficit, but merely serve to describe the child's linguistic functioning.

The other, much more generally favoured, solution (Aarons & Gittens, 1990) would be to call the underlying deficit 'autism' and describe individuals as having degrees and types of this. This may help the child and his family gain access to the support available to those with autism but, as Aarons and Gittens point out, 'the label "autism" has such negative connotations for some clinicians that they are reluctant even to consider it in relation to those children who are less seriously affected'. It is generally agreed, however, that one should not give a linguistic label to avoid having to give the possibly less acceptable diagnosis of autistic disorder.

◯ Identification of Children with Semantic–Pragmatic Disorder

Were these children identified at all 20 years ago? It is possible that their difficulties were misconstrued and thought to be a reflection of more general learning difficulties. Perhaps then they were educated in schools for children with moderate learning difficulties. The difficulties they experienced, especially if misinterpreted or mismanaged, may have led to behavioural difficulties. Rapin and Allen (1983) described a child with Semantic–Pragmatic Syndrome who had severe behavioural problems and was viewed as psychotic, his problems resembling childhood schizophrenia. Certain children may therefore have attended schools catering for behavioural problems.

Were these children referred to speech and language therapy? Perhaps not, but, as speech and language therapists have given more attention to pragmatic functioning, referrals have increased. Those referring clients to speech and language therapy are now more aware of communication impairments dealt with by therapists.

Nowadays we should attempt to identify children's semantic and pragmatic problems. We should also hope that, if these are the primary cause of their inability to access the curriculum, they are in the correct educational setting, which is one that understands and caters for their special educational needs.

◯ Summary

Children have semantic, pragmatic and other linguistic impairments for a variety of reasons. We need to take a holistic, multiprofessional approach when assessing a child with any type of developmental disorder to identify his specific difficulties. This will guarantee the correct educational and general support systems for the child and his family.

In certain cases there may be some justification in labelling the child's linguistic deficits only (for instance when a child has a word-finding difficulty affecting pragmatic skills). Otherwise, Semantic–Pragmatic Disorder should be accepted as a descriptive linguistic label that usually applies (to some degree) to any child with a central processing disorder.

Although displaying the range of difficulties associated with this disorder, certain children may have the most significant deficits in linguistic areas. However, if a 'diagnosis' of Semantic–Pragmatic Disorder is then given, we should recognize the common underlying cognitive disorder that most of these children share with those with autism or Asperger Syndrome. This is especially the case if we wish to plan appropriate intervention based on a true understanding of the child's difficulties.

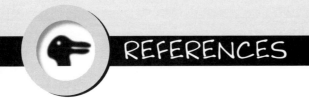

REFERENCES

Aarons M & Gittens T, 'What is the true essence of Autism?', *Speech Therapy in Practice* 5:8, 1990.

Adams C & Bishop DV 'Conversational characteristics of children with semantic–pragmatic disorder I: Exchange structure, turntaking, repairs and cohesion', *British Journal of Disorders of Communication* 24, pp211–239, 1989.

Amery H & Cartwright S, *First 100 Words*, Usbourne, 1987.

Amery H & Cartwright S, *First Thousand Words*, Usbourne, 1995.

Bishop DV & Adams C, 'Conversational characteristics of children with semantic-pragmatic disorder I: Exchange structure, turntaking, repairs and cohesion', *British Journal of Disorders of Communication* 24, pp211-239, 1989.

Bishop DV & Adams C, 'Comprehension problems in children with specific language impairment: literal and inferential meaning', *Journal of Speech and Hearing Research* 35, pp119–129, 1992.

Bishop DVM 'Autism, Asperger's syndrome and semantic–pragmatic disorder: Where are the boundaries?', *British Journal of Disorders of Communication* 24, pp107–121, 1989.

Blank M, Gessner M & Esposito A, 'Language without communication: A case study', *Journal of Child Language* 6, pp329–352, 1979.

Boucher J, 'SPD as a distinct diagnostic entity: logical considerations and directions for future research', *International Journal of Language and Communication Disorders* 33, pp71–81, 1998.

Brook SL & Bowler DM, 'Autism by Another Name? Semantic and Pragmatic Impairments in Children', *Journal of Autism and Developmental Disorders* 22, pp61–81, 1992.

Cromer RF, 'Developmental Language Disorders: Cognitive Processes, Semantics, Pragmatics, Phonology and Syntax', *Journal of Autism and Developmental Disorders* 11, pp57–73, 1981.

Crystal D, *A Dictionary of Linguistics and Phonetics*, Blackwell, Oxford, 1985.

Culloden M, Hyde-Wright S & Shipman A, 'Non-syntactic features of "semantic–pragmatic" disorders', *Advances in working with language disordered children*, ICAN, London, 1986.

Frith U, *Autism: Explaining the Enigma*, Blackwell, Oxford, 1989.

Gagnon L, Mottron L & Joanette Y, 'Questioning the validity of the semantic pragmatic syndrome diagnosis', *Autism* 1, pp37–55, 1997.

Hockey V, 'How to diagnose the child with "HLLD"', *Speech Therapy in Practice* 5:7, 1989.

Jarrold C, Boucher J & Russell J, 'Language profiles in children with autism: theoretical and methodological implications', *Autism* 1, pp57–76, 1997.

Jones S, Smedley M & Jennings M, 'Case study: A child with a high level language disorder characterised by syntactic, semantic and pragmatic difficulties', *Papers in Advances in Working with Language Disordered Children*, 17–21, ICAN, London, 1986.

Kanner L, 'Autistic disturbances of affective contact', *The Nervous Child* 2, pp217–250, 1943.

Kanner L, 'Irrelevant and metaphorical language in early infantile autism', *American Journal of Psychiatry* 103, pp242–246, 1946.

Kerbel D & Grunwell P, 'A study of idiom comprehension in children with semantic–pragmatic difficulties. Part II: Between-groups results and discussion', *International Journal of Language and Communication Disorders* 33, pp23–44, 1998.

Kerbel D, Grunwell P & Grundy K, 'A play-based methodology for assessing idiom comprehension in children with semantic–pragmatic difficulties', *European Journal of Disorders of Communication* 31, pp65–75, 1996.

Paul R, 'Communication', Cohen D, Donnellan A & Paul R (eds), *Handbook of Autism and Pervasive Developmental Disorders*, Wiley, New York, 1987.

Rapin I & Allen D, 'Developmental language disorders: nosologic consideration', Kirk U (ed), *Neuropsychology of Language Reading and Spelling*, Academic Press, New York, 1983.

Rapin I & Allen D, 'The semantic–pragmatic deficit disorder: classification issues', *International Journal of Language and Communication Disorders* 33, pp82–87, 1998.

Shields J, Varley R, Broks P & Simpson A, 'Hemispheric Function in Developmental Language Disorders & High Level Autism', *Developmental Medicine and Child Neurology* 38, pp473–486, 1996.

Wing L 'The Continuum of autistic characteristics', Schopler E & Mealbous GB (eds), *Diagnosis and Assessment in Autism*, Plenum, New York, 1988.

Also available from Speechmark

Working with Pragmatics

Lucie Andersen-Wood & Benita Rae Smith

Contains practical pragmatic teaching activities to develop communication skills. Offers an opportunity to explore this subject with confidence and to plan intervention programmes for effective management. Photocopiable assessment forms are included.

Autism: A social skills approach for children & adolescents

Maureen Aarons & Tessa Gittens

An excellent source of practical ideas on which to base programmes of intervention for children with autism. The content is primarily aimed at those working with children who have normal, or near normal, cognitive abilities, rather than those whose autism accompanies severe learning disabilities.

PETAL. Phonological Evaluation & Transcription of Audio-Visual Language

Anne Parker

PETAL is a tool for describing speech production patterns of children and adults in relationship to factors which may enhance or impede speech intelligibility. The approach used was originally developed for use with deaf children and adults, where the need to take account of audible and visible factors in speech assessment, development and conversation is a key factor. This boxed set includes photocopiable resources and 10 sets of illustrated cards.

Children's Phonology Sourcebook

Lesley Flynn & Gwen Lancaster

Lively and entertaining practical resource materials for speech and language therapists and others who work with young speech-disordered children can be found in this Winslow manual. Linking theory to practice, this is a user-friendly resource which encourages a thoughtful and creative approach to language remediation work.

Working with Children's Phonology

Gwen Lancaster & Lesley Pope

Successfully bridging the gap between theory and practice, this unique manual provides numerous creative ideas for lively and entertaining activities. It is a stimulating and essential resource which emphasises clinical approaches, contains clearly presented concepts, includes well illustrated original activities and examines advances in the analysis and description of phonological disorders.

Working with Children's Language

Jackie Cooke & Diana Williams

Well established and ever popular, this leading manual provides countless ideas along with a huge range of activities for language teaching. The combination of games, activities and ideas for developing specific language skills contribute to making this handbook a valuable resource for everyone working with children.

Early Communication Skills
New Revised Edition

Charlotte Lynch & Julia Cooper

Containing a wealth of communication based activities, this practical resource will be invaluable to all professionals looking for fresh educational and therapeutic ideas in their work with preschool children and their parents.

Early Listening Skills

Diana Williams

This is a highly practical and user-friendly activity manual for professionals working with pre-school children who have underdeveloped listening skills associated with language delay, hearing loss or other communication difficulty.

Early Sensory Skills

Jackie Cooke

Creating a compendium of practical and enjoyable activities for vision, touch, taste and smell, this photocopiable manual is an invaluable resource for anyone working with children. The author outlines major principles and aims in six easy-to-use sections containing basic activities, everyday activities, games and topics to stimulate and develop the senses.

These are just a few of the many therapy resources available from Speechmark. A free catalogue will be sent on request. For further information please contact:

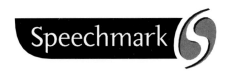

Telford Road • Bicester • Oxon OX26 4LQ • UK
Telephone: (01869) 244644
Facsimile: (01869) 320040
www.speechmark.net

Semantic-Pragmatic
LANGUAGE DISORDER

Charlotte Firth

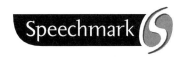

Speechmark

Telford Road • Bicester • Oxon OX26 4LQ • UK

Editor's Note

For the sake of clarity alone, in this pack we have used 'he' to refer to the child.

Published by
Speechmark Publishing Ltd, Telford Road, Bicester, Oxon OX26 4LQ
United Kingdom
www.speechmark.net

002-3342/Printed in the United Kingdom/1030
British Library Cataloguing in Publication Data
Firth, Charlotte,
    Photocopiable guide, checklists & therapy ideas
    Part 2 Charlotte Firth, Katherine Venkatesh
    1. Speech disorders in children 2. Speech disorders in children – Diagnosis
    3. Speech therapy for children
    I. Title II. Venkatesh, Katherine
    618.9'2855'06

ISBN for Part 2: 0 86388 327 3
ISBN for complete set of 3 volumes: ISBN 0 86388 329 X
ISBN for Part 1: 0 86388 326 5
ISBN for Part 3: 0 86388 328 1
Previously published by Winslow Press Ltd under ISBN 0 86388 240 4 (Part 1),
0 86388 241 2 (Part 2), 0 86388 242 0 (Part 3), 0 86388 203 X (complete set)

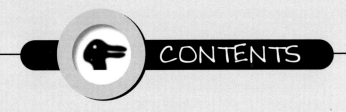

CONTENTS

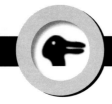

QUESTIONS & ANSWERS

A guide to the disorder for parents & teachers

Section 2

QUESTIONS & ANSWERS

This section has been designed to be photocopied and handed to parents and teachers

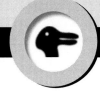

QUESTIONS & ANSWERS

○ What do 'Semantic' and 'Pragmatic' Mean?

'Semantic' and 'Pragmatic' are linguistic terms. 'Semantics' is the study of words and their meanings. Children change and sort out the meaning of words as they make concepts about the world around them. A young child may learn that his pet cat is called 'Tom' and then call all small animals 'Toms'. However, as a child experiences more situations and talks about them, he starts to understand how, for instance, a 'Tom' differs from a rabbit and he may then understand and use 'cat'. A child at this stage has some concept of his surroundings and appreciates the concept of 'animal'. He would not say a rabbit was a 'lorry'.

As classifications and relationships between items begin to be further understood, the child selects words based on this knowledge. For example, as a child begins to understand the concept of position, words such as 'on' and 'behind' start to develop and when children start to see how different actions vary and are classified, verbs develop in their speech. Semantic development therefore relies on a child's ability to reason, understand and subsequently make concepts about his world.

Pragmatics is the study of the way language (verbal and non-verbal) is used to interact with others in social situations. Communication does not rely only on words. Babies start to communicate very early: they soon learn that crying can gain the attention of their carers. Babies also have 'conversations' with other people, using eye contact, cooing and, later, babble sequences in a turn-taking routine to 'talk'.

As speech develops, children build on these communication skills and use words in a variety of ways, for instance to question, give instructions or describe. At an early language stage, one word, such as 'car', can be given different meanings by the child using a variety of intonation patterns: for instance, "car?" ("Is this a car?") or "car!" ("I want a car"). Gradually children develop and refine their ability to be involved in conversation and use language appropriate to different contexts. Children still developing these skills may still shout, "Mummy, look at that lady's funny hat!", but gradually, through an appreciation of the thoughts and feelings of other people and a natural readiness to relate to others, more appropriate pragmatic skills develop.

What May Cause Semantic and Pragmatic Language Difficulties?

Children may have difficulties in these areas for several reasons, including the following:

1 A child with a hearing impairment may find it difficult to develop a vocabulary as quickly as children with adequate hearing. He may not be able to gain the same amount from everyday situations as other children. A child with a hearing loss may also find it hard to follow and join in conversation.

2 Children with articulation or speech sound difficulties may appear to be using incorrect words or may choose to use words that they know they can articulate. They may also appreciate that they often fail to make themselves understood and consequently may avoid talking to others. They may then have real difficulties in conversation when they try.

3 Children with problems understanding spoken language may have delayed vocabulary (and grammatical) abilities and are consequently likely to find it hard to converse with adults and friends.

4 Children with an expressive language disorder (who may find it hard to construct a sentence or remember words) are again likely to have problems using appropriate words in their speech, and following normal conversational rules. (**NB** This group of children are often confused with children with a 'true' semantic–pragmatic disorder: see below.)

However, although speech and language difficulties such as those above can cause semantic and pragmatic problems, most children whose language disorder is labelled 'semantic–pragmatic' have a particular type of difficulty. This particular problem affects the way they develop and acquire abilities generally, not just in their language skills.

We all sense things in our surroundings, such as what we see, feel, taste and so on. We then absorb this information and use it to reason, make concepts and rationalize about what we are experiencing. In this way we are able to learn from experiences. However, certain children seem to be over- or undersensitive to the things they experience. This may be because they seem to find it hard to process what they experience using their knowledge of similar situations.

As a result, a child with this type of problem will find it hard to deal with new situations and will only feel secure and happy with, for instance, well known sounds, tastes, situations and people. It will be difficult for him to infer and consequently to rationalize in any new situation and this can then be upsetting for him. (For instance, he may cover his ears at certain noises or throw a tantrum if someone new visits his home.) A child with this type of difficulty will develop vocabulary skills, but words are mainly learnt and memorized and not built up on a basis of a developing ability to make concepts about the world. Because of this, semantic skills are affected. In addition, a child who has difficulty making sense of his world in this way may find it hard to interpret the thoughts and feelings of others and consequently find people confusing and difficult to deal with. He will then prefer his own company or may have problems understanding and dealing with the rules of interaction.

What are the Significant Characteristics of a Semantic–Pragmatic Language Disorder?

Children with a semantic–pragmatic language disorder appear to have a significant degree of difficulty processing information in the ways already discussed. This affects how their linguistic skills develop in certain characteristic ways. There is a predictable pattern to the development of their verbal and non-verbal skills, which may be simplified into four stages (ages given are approximate).

Stage 1 Birth to Age 2

Communication skills

It is unlikely that a communication disorder would be recognized in a very young baby, but parents of children with a semantic–pragmatic disorder often comment that their child was an undemanding baby and was quite passive. He may have cried if in discomfort or when hungry, but not for attention. He may not have enjoyed eye contact with others or engaged in early cooing and babble turn-taking sequences to converse. He may also have been unwilling to join in with 'peek-a-boo' or other such games.

Other areas

Parents may also remember that even as a baby their child was upset by changes in routine, or by unfamiliar places or people. For instance, he may only have liked to be picked up by certain people. Weaning can be one of the first major changes in a baby's life and babies with this disorder sometimes resist this change.

Often parents cite a particular event as the origin of their child's difficulties, saying, for example, "He was all right until .... " It may not have been the actual event that *caused* the difficulties, however; rather the event made the underlying problem (lack of acceptance of change) more apparent.

Stage 2 Age 3 to 5

Communication skills

Children usually start to develop spoken language at around nine to 18 months. As mentioned before, the development of vocabulary and grammatical skills is based mainly on an ability to make concepts about the world. As this happens, words and phrases of increasing complexity are generated.

2

As well as this, children also remember whole phrases without usually understanding every word in them. It seems that children with a semantic–pragmatic language disorder mainly use this latter method. They use their often very good memory to remember speech, but do not gradually develop their ability to generate or build up phrases. Remembering phrases rather than generating them is a difficult way to learn language, and communication difficulties are sometimes suspected at this age as the child may be late to speak.

Often at this stage the child will echo what he has heard, perhaps as a way of committing to memory whatever someone has said. He may also do this because he has not understood what has been said and is therefore just 'bouncing it back'. Certain very regular sequences of language are often remembered especially well, for instance the alphabet or numbers. It is not always apparent, however, that the child has difficulty understanding speech — even the speech he uses himself.

Conversations are difficult at this stage as the child may prefer his own company and may only use speech for his own enjoyment (for instance, he may recite learnt phrases but not use these a great deal to relate to others). The child may seem to talk *at* you, rather than *with* you.

Other areas

By this stage a child with a semantic–pragmatic disorder may have developed certain strong likes and dislikes which may not be very apparent until he is exposed to new experiences, such as going to a playgroup. A child who has difficulty making sense of the world will feel more secure and happy with familiar situations such as those at home.

He may have a certain restricted range of foods he will eat, certain videos he will watch (often over and over again) or toys with which he will play (often in a particular set way). In addition, he may not play in a make-believe way, though he may 'play' as he has been taught to or act out scenes from favourite books or videos.

Stage 3 — Age 6 to 8

Communication Skills

Often by this stage children with Semantic–Pragmatic Disorder appear to have good language skills. They may produce well formed sentences. They may also have quite complex words in their vocabulary that can astound the listener. These skills can mask underlying difficulties as the child may still have problems understanding language and concepts.

He may favour particular topics and talk about these without any appreciation of the actual topic of conversation in hand. Often speech is repetitive; for instance, he may ask questions over and over again without any real interest in the answer (this is probably because he enjoys the predictable nature of your response).

In addition, the child tends to be insensitive to the needs of his conversational partners. He may talk at the same time as the other person or direct a monologue at them. The child's speech also varies in its appropriateness, from being totally out of context to being just slightly odd; for instance, "It's going to rain" when it is actually raining.

At this stage poor body language may become more apparent: he may face away from you when talking. Other non-verbal aspects of language can also be a problem for the child. For instance, he may not appreciate how tone of voice can alter the meaning of something. Therefore, because the child has learnt whole phrases together with a particular intonation pattern he may not use the correct intonation when repeating the phrase in a particular situation. He may also use a certain set intonation pattern when talking.

The child with semantic–pragmatic language disorder will be increasing his ability to interpret language by this stage. He may, however, be in the rather unusual position of being able to say much more than he can understand. Consequently, adults may direct quite complex language at the child and conversation can break down. Although the child can produce a considerable amount of speech by this stage, he often has great problems when trying to say something specific about a new situation (for instance, in response to a Speech & Language Therapist's test pictures).

Once a child has lots of memorized language, he may try to use 'chunks' of these phrases to try to say something more appropriate. As a result, sentences can then appear slightly odd or misformulated, as with "The dog is barking to chase the cat." In addition, he may struggle to remember learnt phrases and words, and have 'false starts' when starting to explain or describe something, for example, "put it, pu put to, put it to the chair, **on** the chair".

Another characteristic feature often apparent at this stage is confusion over the use of suitable names and pronouns. People may say "Peter" in connection with a child and he may go on to refer to himself in that way, as in "Peter is tired" (that is, "I am tired"). He may hear everyone call his parents by their first names and consequently use these names in connection with his parents, not 'Mum' and 'Dad'. The child may also refer to himself as 'you', as this is what other people say in connection with him. All this is probably because language is learnt but not altered in relation to the viewpoint of the speaker.

Other areas
Almost obsessive interests may develop in certain, often repetitive, predictable subjects as the child will feel comfortable and reassured by well

known things. Some children with Semantic–Pragmatic Disorder have certain movements they make when they are anxious or excited, such as hand flapping, perhaps again for reassurance.

Because he has a good auditory and visual memory, a child may learn to read with relative ease, but he may not always understand what he has read. At this stage the child may still be upset by changes in routine, and starting school can be a very disturbing time, making him very anxious.

Stage ④ Age 9 and Above

Communication skills

As the child matures he is expected to appreciate the increasingly subtle ways language is used in different contexts. Children with a Semantic–Pragmatic Disorder tend to continue to interpret language in a very concrete way and consequently speech is taken very literally. Areas such as humour, sarcasm and metaphor, as in, "Pull your socks up!" may therefore create confusion and very strange reactions!

He may not make inferences about a situation or the people in it. For instance, if asked "Can you turn the page?", he may answer, "Yes" but not act on it. Because of this, those who do not understand the nature if the child's problems may misconstrue his behaviour as rude. For instance, of he is warned, "Do that one more time" he may interpret this as an instruction and do it.

Conversational skills continue to be unusual and he may need to be taught more appropriate rules of discourse. He may still find other people slightly confusing but, if motivated, can be helped to work out what others are probably thinking and feeling. Without these skills he may say too much or too little: for example, "I bought a new one there" (without saying to what 'one' and 'there' relate). At this stage the child may still have difficulties taking turns in conversation. He may also talk excessively about a particular subject, without realizing it may be boring to the listener. In addition, the child may use inappropriate volume and/or tone of voice when talking. His speech can also appear too adult and overly precise.

Other areas

Older children with a Semantic–Pragmatic Disorder can sometimes experience difficulties at school as tasks are presented in more abstract ways, using more complex language and possibly fewer visual cues. Secondary education can pose extra problems as the child then has to deal with different lessons, teachers, rooms and complex timetables (and each teacher will have a slightly different linguistic style). Identification of the child's difficulties is very important as they may not be particularly obvious by this stage.

○ What is the Relationship to Autism?

Parents of children with a semantic–pragmatic language disorder may hear about children with autism and see similarities between their child and the children being described. Perhaps their child has been described as having 'autistic features' or 'tendencies'. Whether a semantic–pragmatic language disorder is the same as, related to, or similar to autism has been the topic of many discussions.

Perhaps we should look at the underlying disorder. This difficulty means certain individuals process and integrate sensory information in ways that are significantly unusual and this affects the way they develop and acquire skills in certain areas. This problem can vary from a severe to a very mild impairment and may then create varying degrees of difficulties in a number of different developmental areas.

When this sensory processing difficulty has the most significant effect on *language* development, it may be most helpful to describe the child's disorder in linguistic terms. He may have other developmental problems, but to a less significant degree. We could then use the label, 'semantic–pragmatic disorder'. We should still appreciate, however, that the child has, to some degree, the same underlying problem as a child with autism. A person with autism *is* likely to have a pragmatic disorder. This may not be the most pertinent area or problem to label, however, given the more severe level of the additional difficulties that person has in other areas (such as with social functioning).

It could be argued that everyone falling within this spectrum of disorders should be described as being mildly to severely 'autistic'.

Another view is that 'autism' should be a label for a particular type and degree of the underlying disorder. If we take this view, to describe a child with a Semantic–Pragmatic Disorder as being 'mildly autistic' or as having 'autistic features' would be the same as describing someone who is short-sighted as being 'mildly blind' or having 'blindness features'. However, we do need to be aware if the child has semantic and pragmatic difficulties as a result of his condition being within the range of disorders that includes autism. If we do not address this question we may miss the true nature of the child's difficulties.

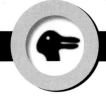

PROBLEMS & SOLUTIONS

The difficulties children & parents encounter with this type of language disorder, and some helpful strategies

PROBLEMS & SOLUTIONS

This section has been designed to be photocopied and handed to parents and teachers

PROBLEMS & SOLUTIONS

○ Common difficulties and possible solutions

Listed below are some of the characteristic difficulties that children with this type of disorder often encounter. The points are arranged in chronological order, working from features seen in the younger child to those more characteristic of the older child.

THE CHILD • *May be distressed by changes in his environment.*

HOW YOU CAN HELP • Remain alert to even the most subtle changes, for instance wearing a new perfume or following a different routine when out shopping.

THE CHILD • *May carry out repetitive movements.*

HOW YOU CAN HELP • Do not try to stop the child. Be aware that they may make him feel less anxious as they are familiar and predictable.

THE CHILD • *May become upset by new people and situations.*

HOW YOU CAN HELP • Explain, in very simple language, what is going to happen. For example, "A lady is coming to see you; she will talk to you, then she will go." If you think it 'goes without saying', it probably does not!

THE CHILD • *May be uninterested in interaction.*

HOW YOU CAN HELP • Be aware that he may find people hard to cope with and prefer his own company. Try to increase his tolerance of you, however, by playing alongside him and gradually intervening in his activities.

THE CHILD • *May show little interest in using babble to 'chat' with.*

HOW YOU CAN HELP • Copy sounds the child makes and/or give him a favourite toy as he makes the sound.

THE CHILD • *May be keen to learn words that are not terribly useful in everyday life, such as 'penguins'!*

HOW YOU CAN HELP • First, try to make these words work for the child, for instance, produce a few zoo animals if your child says this word. Always try to work from this to emphasize more functional words, such as body parts of the animals.

THE CHILD • *May be late to start talking.*

HOW YOU CAN HELP • Be aware that the child may not be learning to talk in the usual way. His method may be mainly to memorize words. He has to get to a certain developmental stage before he starts doing this.

THE CHILD • *May be eager to repeat the things you say.*

HOW YOU CAN HELP • This can be rather annoying. Remember that the child is either doing this to memorize what you have said so he can also say it (be careful what you say!) or he may be echoing because he has not understood you.

THE CHILD • *May find it hard to understand speech.*

HOW YOU CAN HELP • Remember that the child may have a good memory, but may not fully understand all the words and phrases he has memorized. Warn others to use simple speech when talking to him.

THE CHILD • *May become obsessed with certain books, toys or videos.*

HOW YOU CAN HELP • Recognize that the child likes familiar, predictable, regular things as these give him something that he can rely on in a world that often seems rather confusing and unpredictable. Again, try to build activities from his interests, but do not deny him them altogether as this will make him very anxious and unable to cope with anything else presented.

THE CHILD • *May talk a great deal, perhaps to himself, but not use speech to converse with.*

HOW YOU CAN HELP • Try to make him use his speech to ask for things, give you instructions and so on. Although he may learn to recite language quite easily (he may count, say the alphabet or tell you the characters from *Thomas the Tank Engine*) remember that these are not very useful in conversation.

THE CHILD • *May find it difficult to 'process' incoming information: things he sees, feels, tastes, hears and smells.*

HOW YOU CAN HELP • Be aware that certain sensations may upset the child. A new jumper may feel too rough or a sound that you hardly notice may bother the child quite considerably. Try to work out what seemingly inconsequential thing may be upsetting him if he becomes distressed.

THE CHILD • *May go on to understand language quite well 'on the surface'.*

HOW YOU CAN HELP • Although he may seem to understand, be aware that misunderstandings can occur. For instance, if you say, "Peter, throw the dice," do not get cross if he does just that. The child may have difficulties appreciating how words differ in their meaning according to the context.

THE CHILD • *May go on to produce rather 'adult-like' speech.*

HOW YOU CAN HELP • Remember that he has memorized speech he has heard. Appreciate also that this is not necessarily a good thing. *You* may be impressed with his extensive vocabulary and complex phrases, but his peers will not be! Encourage him to use speech characteristic of a child of his age to help him socialize.

THE CHILD • *May use language repetitively, for instance to ask lots of questions.*

HOW YOU CAN HELP • Again, this is because the child likes familiar things. A certain question is likely to get a particular answer and is therefore predictable. However, this can become rather annoying, so answer the child but warn him that you may not answer again, or say, "You know the answer to that, Peter." Tell him it is annoying!

THE CHILD • *May have poor conversational skills.*

HOW YOU CAN HELP • Do not forget that he may find it hard to 'read into' situations and the people in them. He will find it hard to know when to join in a conversation and know what to say. Congratulate him if, for example, he listens to what has been said, but inform him of the rules if he gets it wrong: for instance, "Wait until the other person has finished speaking before you speak." Again, state the obvious.

THE CHILD • *May monopolise conversations with long monologues.*

HOW YOU CAN HELP • The child may enjoy speaking for speaking's sake and not be interested in your responses. Try to interject by asking questions or giving information that relates to his topic. Let him know that it is usual to do this in conversation.

THE CHILD • *May change topic frequently.*

HOW YOU CAN HELP • Explain to the child what he has done. Say "You have started to talk about… we were talking about… we'll go back to that later". Then carry on with the existing topic. You could work on ways of introducing new ideas, for instance phrases such as, "Oh, by the way …"

THE CHILD • *May ignore your questions and give an irrelevant response.*

HOW YOU CAN HELP • The child may find it hard to process question forms. Use other cues such as pointing and gesture to help him. If you feel he has just ignored your question and is saying whatever comes to mind, then keep repeating whatever you said until he 'tunes in' to you.

THE CHILD • *May have difficulties interpreting facial expression and tone of voice.*

HOW YOU CAN HELP • Do not expect him to pick up subtle cues: "Simon!", said in a 'do that one more time and you're in big trouble', way, may mean nothing to him. He may just wonder why you are saying his name. Similarly, do not expect him to fully interpret your facial expression. This, with the verbal comprehension difficulties, can mean that his behaviour can be construed as rather naughty. For instance, imagine that, if you say, "How many times do I have to tell you?," he may enquire "Five?".

THE CHILD • *May have difficulties with metaphor and other non-literal language.*

HOW YOU CAN HELP • Be aware of how much language is metaphorical. Phrases like 'Pull your socks up' are obviously open to misconception, but what about "Tell me a number *bigger* than ten", or "Do it in your head"? You may have to analyse what you have said if the child does or says something very odd.

THE CHILD • *May not see himself as part of a group.*

HOW YOU CAN HELP • Appreciate that the child may not realize that instructions given to the group he is in actually apply to him. You may need to say his name or get his attention specifically, before saying what to do: for instance, not "Right, everyone go outside now" but "*John*, go outside now!"

THE CHILD • *May need a routine.*

HOW YOU CAN HELP • Be aware that certain things do have quite a set pattern, as with the school day/week. More unusual events, such as Christmas activities, a photographer visiting or a school trip, can disrupt this routine. Warn the child in advance, explain what will happen and when things will be back to normal.

THE CHILD • *May have problems when trying to explain things.*

HOW YOU CAN HELP • Don't forget that, even when the child has a lot of language, he will not find it easy to explain very specific events as he will have to *formulate* phrases, rather than just using memorized language. Give him time to try to sort out what he is saying. Sometimes it might help to repeat what he has said, but in a coherent way. Then he has a good model if he needs to express something similar in the future.

THE CHILD • *May seem to read well.*

HOW YOU CAN HELP • Remember that the child may be using his good (visual) memory. He may enjoy racing through his reading books and schemes, but may not understand most of what he has read. He will need lots of comprehension work. Also try to make reading functional, for instance by looking at food packets or information leaflets which he may be interested in.

THE CHILD • *May give too little information: for instance, "Ours is called Sidney and it's in the big one." (When you have no idea who Sidney might be and what is big.)*

HOW YOU CAN HELP • You must for example, explain, to the child that he has not said what 'it' is and that you do not know what he is referring to. Ask for more information, then point out where his information was lacking. For instance: "Oh, you've got a rabbit. I didn't know that because I haven't been to your house." "Have I seen your garden?" (No) "Then how could I have known that you had a big and a little shed?"

THE CHILD • *May use inappropriate speech 'codes', for instance, he may talk too casually or too formally in a given situation.*

HOW YOU CAN HELP • Give the child a more appropriate model, explain what would be appropriate in that situation. For instance, if he says, "Hiya, Mr Thompson, what did you have for breakfast?", say, "No, we don't say that ... just say, 'Good morning Mr. Thompson'."

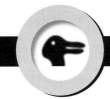

CHECKLIST A

A developmental checklist
in four stages:
0–2 years; 3–5 years;
6–8 years; 9 years and above

Section

4

CHECKLIST A

**This Checklist should be
photocopied by the clinician
for use with parents or carers**

CHECKLIST A

○ Checklist A

Some of the features described in this checklist are evident when many children communicate. However, those with a semantic–pragmatic disorder will usually display most of the characteristics. Each stage gives approximate age levels. Complete those stages up to and including the age of the child at assessment. Score one for each tick.

A suggested score is given at the end of each stage. The child should achieve this score, or higher, in the stage he is at *and* in the preceding stages. If the child achieves the suggested score, this could indicate a semantic–pragmatic language disorder.

Choose the stage that describes the child most effectively at the time of assessment and cross-refer to the therapy ideas for that stage in Section 6.

4

Undemanding of social interaction or 'company' as a baby.

☐

Often described as a very good baby.

☐

Uninterested in eye contact with carer.

☐

Lack of interest in early turn-taking games, such as 'peek-a-boo'.

☐

May not use vocalizations to hold a 'conversation'.

☐

Distressed by weaning or other significant changes, such as the birth of a sibling.

☐

People may say, "He was all right until ..."

☐

Distressed by changes in his environment.

☐

Unhappy in the company of unfamiliar people.

☐

May exhibit repetitive movements, such as hand flapping, when excited or anxious.

☐

Little or no babble used.

☐

Suggested score **8** **Child's score** ☐

P

4

First words may be late. ☐

First words may be unusual, eg. 'hedgehog' (may be related to the child's interests). ☐

Restricted diet. ☐

Echoes what has been said. (By end of this stage he may be echoing almost silently.) ☐

Moves quickly from little or no speech to using long phrases. ☐

Enjoys rough-and-tumble play but not light physical contact. ☐

Strong interest in certain toys, books or videos. ☐

Good memory (auditory and visual) becomes evident. ☐

Memorizes and overuses certain phrases. ☐

Poor symbolic play, may learn certain routines with toys. ☐

Poor ability to understand speech. (Parents/carers may suspect he cannot hear or does not listen.) ☐

Certain sounds may distress the child; he may cover his ears. ☐

Recites language, but does not *use* speech to communicate in a variety of ways. ☐

Feels safer with certain known routines; becomes distressed in new situations. ☐

Finds it hard to respond appropriately to questions. ☐

Appears to have become less anxious, but new experiences such as starting school may upset him. ☐

Asks questions with little regard to answers. ☐

Suggested score **13**   **Child's score** ☐

Stage 3 **6 – 8 YEARS**

Copes relatively well with standardized speech and language assessments, but has difficulty with more abstract language. ☐

Can probably say more than he can understand. ☐

Has learnt concrete concepts but in a rigid way, perhaps relating to therapy materials. ☐

May change the subject in conversation without warning. ☐

May have difficulty with temporal concepts and associated language (May misuse 'tomorrow', 'next', 'after' and so on.) ☐

Produces seemingly well formed sentences (perhaps a little too 'adult-like' or precise). ☐

Favours particular topics and quite often leads the conversation round to these. ☐

Uses repetitive language; for instance, may ask many questions, with little interest in the answers. ☐

Talks 'over' you; poor at turn taking. ☐

Says irrelevant or inappropriate things. ☐

Has word-finding problems; may select words incorrectly. ☐

Inappropriate body language; for instance, may face or look away. ☐

Still echoes speech, but in a slightly more appropriate way; for instance: "Would you like a biscuit now?" "Like a biscuit now!" ☐

May use neologisms (eg. 'Slicket'). ☐

Uses unusual intonation patterns (tone of voice): for instance, very jerky speech or rising tones on every phrase. ☐

Dominates play sessions; may not be open to ideas of peers. ☐

Sentences may appear slightly odd or misformulated, especially when he is trying to explain something new. ☐

When starting to say something may have 'false starts': for instance, "I, I had, I have a … ". ☐

Has difficulty with personal pronouns, may use 'you' to refer to himself or his name rather than 'I' or 'me'. ☐

Uses other pronouns as heard; for example, says "Put *your* coat on", meaning, "Help me put *my* coat on." ☐

May still have strong interests and definite likes and dislikes. ☐

Owing to a good memory for what has been heard and seen, he may learn to read quickly but may find it harder to *understand* written material. ☐

Repetitive movements begin to diminish. ☐

May have difficulty interpreting tone of voice and facial expression.
(Can cause difficulties in class.) ☐

Does not see himself as part of a group. ☐

May engage in eye contact but in an unusual way, may seem to 'look through you' for instance. ☐

Suggested score 20   **Child's score** ☐

Interprets language in very literal ways. ☐

Difficulties inferring, that is, working out what people actually *mean* by what they say. ☐

He may launch into long monologues, without any awareness of how the listener is responding. ☐

Gives information that is not needed; for instance, may state what colour items are. ☐

May have difficulties using referential terms; that is, may say, "The man is walking and the man is wearing a coat" (rather than ".... and *he* is wearing ..."). ☐

May have difficulties establishing referents, for instance, uses words such as 'it' without informing you what 'it' is. ☐

May have difficulties understanding humorous language, sarcasm, metaphor, similes and so on. ☐

Has difficulty working out what others know and may be thinking. ☐

May not use appropriate speech 'code'; for instance, may talk too casually to a teacher or in a formal way to peers. ☐

May want to make friends, but attempts often fail. Peers may find him annoying or irritating. ☐

Continues to have difficulties interpreting non-verbal aspects of language. ☐

Accepts a more varied diet. ☐

Enjoys slapstick humour. ☐

Has word-finding difficulties. ☐

Lacks confidence in social situations. ☐

Easily led when with peers; naive, may get into trouble unwittingly. ☐

May want to join in conversations, but attempts often fail. ☐

May have very rigid opinions, may find it hard to be flexible in response to a particular situation. ☐

Suggested score 14   **Child's score** ☐

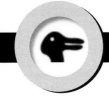

CHECKLIST B

A general informative checklist for parents or carers

Section 5

CHECKLIST B

This Checklist should be photocopied and completed by parents or carers

CHECKLIST B

'Semantic' is a term used to describe how words have meanings. Children build up their understanding and use of words on the basis of a growing understanding of the world around them.

'Pragmatic' language abilities relate to the way language and other, non-verbal, skills (such as tone of voice and facial expression) are used to interact with others in social situations. Children are born with an ability and aptitude to relate to others, and these skills continue to develop into adulthood.

Children with a semantic–pragmatic language disorder have unusual vocabulary skills. They may know a lot about a particular area (such as steam trains) but may not know words that are more useful to them in everyday conversations. A child with a semantic–pragmatic disorder can probably say quite long phrases, but will not use speech to communicate with others in the usual ways.

A child with a semantic–pragmatic language disorder may not do all of the things itemised in the following checklist especially as their difficulties change as they develop. Tick the boxes which refer to your child. If your child exhibits at least half of the features, it is likely he has a communication disability of this type.

Child's Name:
Date this Checklist was completed:
Child's situation:

PLEASE TICK APPROPRIATE BOX

The child may:

have problems speaking at the right time in a conversation and may talk 'over' you at times. ☐

panic in a new situation. ☐

repeat what you have said, at times sounding like an echo. ☐

not follow or remember what you have said. ☐

seem to 'switch off' at times when you are talking. ☐

not play in a 'make-believe' way and just play with a few particular toys, in a certain way, over and over again. ☐

keep changing the subject when you are talking to them. ☐

ask lots of questions, but then not seem very interested in your answers. ☐

give inappropriate answers to your questions. ☐

repeat the same sentence often. ☐

speak at you, rather than talking to you. ☐

not say enough and then expect you to understand what they are talking about. ☐

get muddled up when speaking, especially when starting a sentence. ☐

have certain toys, books or videos with which they are almost 'obsessed'. ☐

like a certain set way of doing things and then get upset if this is changed. ☐

learn to read quite well, but perhaps does not remember or follow what has been read. ☐

understand language in a very literal way. ☐

have problems 'reading between the lines'. For instance, if you say, "Oh no, I've left the door open", he may not realize you would like it to be shut. ☐

have poor eye contact and may even face away from you when talking. ☐

speak too quietly or too loudly. ☐

have an unusual tone of voice when talking. ☐

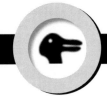

THERAPY IDEAS

Ideas relating to areas of
difficulty detailed in the
four stages of Checklist A

Section 6

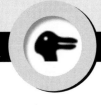

THERAPY IDEAS

Stage 1 0 – 2 YEARS

Children with a semantic–pragmatic language disorder may not develop the usual pre-verbal skills. It may be helpful therefore, even with older children, to encourage these communicative behaviours. Handouts 1 to 8 cover the ideas listed below, but are presented in a more attractive form for parents and carers.

Eye Contact (Handouts 1 & 2)

Eye contact is a very important part of communicating.

- Hold toys up next to your face as you name them: for instance, "look … a car!"

- See if your child notices something silly (a cup, for example) balanced on your head. If not, get him to look at you and to take it off.

- Play peek-a-boo games with your child where you hide your face.

- Put stickers on your nose. Encourage your child to look at you and to pull the stickers off.

- Let your child brush your hair, wash your face, put face paints on you and so on.

Eye contact can also be used to get people's attention.

- Use toys that can be activated such as wind-up toys. When your child looks at the toy and then at you, activate the toy.

- Use bubbles. When your child looks at the container of bubble mixture and then at you, blow some more bubbles.

- At mealtimes have a choice of foods. Encourage your child to choose by looking at the food and then at you.

Pointing (Handout 3)

Pointing helps to communicate our wants and needs.

- Encourage your child to point to things to indicate his preferences. Do this by giving choices at mealtimes, when getting dressed, when playing with toys, and so on.

- Put a favourite toy out of your child's reach. Show your child how to point to it and give the toy to him when he does this.

- Use picture books. Encourage your child to point to the pictures for you to name. When your child makes a recognizable attempt at pointing, name the picture quickly so that he links the two things together.

- When you go out for a walk, encourage your child to point to things he would like to investigate.

Cause & Effect (Handout 4)

In order to communicate we need to understand how to make things happen.

- Choose toys that need switches to activate them, or that make sounds or movements. (for example, Jack-in-the-box, pop-up farm).

- Use your child's vocalizations. When he makes a sound (even if this is not purposeful) give him a toy, food, and so on. See if he starts to realize that sounds can be used to communicate with people.

- Play a game with a doll. Pretending the doll is asleep, say "Shh ... dolly's asleep". Then model getting close to the doll and saying "Boo!!". Make the doll jump and act frightened. Then she goes to sleep again. Can you get your child to say "Boo!" (or any sound initially) as the trigger to wake up the doll?

- Build a tower of bricks and wait for your child to make a sound before teddy knocks it down. You could use this idea with toy cars going down a ramp, or with you kicking a ball.

Making Choices (Handout 5)

Making choices gives your child a chance to communicate his ideas.

- Encourage your child to choose constantly: at mealtimes, when getting dressed, at play. Say, for example, "Do you want milk or orange?", "Shall we give dolly drink or some dinner?" Encourage eye pointing or gesture if your child does not use words.

- In play set up activities for teddy and dolly. Ask, for example, "What shall teddy do now: sleep or jump?"; "Who wants the hat: teddy or dolly?"

- Use an inset puzzle and ask your child to choose which pieces to put back in.

Symbols (Handout 6)

Pictures, toys, drawings and sounds are all symbols for real objects.

- Play object picture matching games. Can your child match objects, first to photographs, then to coloured drawings; then to line drawings?

- Encourage pretend play. First, you and your child act out everyday situations. Then try sequences with dolls and toys (getting up, getting dressed, and so on.) Finally, work towards using small doll's houses and similar toys.

- Your child may try to act out scenes from favourite books or videos and use these characters. Try to develop this into more make-believe play by bringing in other elements, such as animals, people or situations.

- Encourage your child to draw simple line drawings, such as faces or people. Talk through them as you draw together.

- Accompany play with sound effects, such as 'brrm' for cars, noises for animals and so on.

Joint Activities (Handout 7)

Playing with others is one of the first steps towards communication.

- Play joint action games, such as 'Row, row, row your boat …'

- Play finger rhymes such as 'Round and round the garden'. Watch out for your child trying to initiate these games if he enjoys them, for example by holding out his hand.

- In a group everyone has a cup. One person has small beads or bricks in theirs (or water if you are feeling brave!). This person pours the beads or bricks into the next person's cup, who then pours them into the next, and so on. This is more difficult if you can only use one hand, as this requires more joint attention.

- Use construction toys. Join in with your child as he makes a simple model. As he becomes used to this, give more direct suggestions.

- Sit facing your child. Use cars, a ball, wheeled toys and so on to push/roll to each other. You or your child could say "Go!" to get the other person to push the toy.

Turn Taking (Handout 8)

Turn taking is the basis of two-way interaction.

- Build a tower, taking turns to add the bricks.

- Take turns threading large beads onto a string.

- Use pairs of noisemakers … (shakers, tambourines, drums). Take turns making sounds. For example, your child bangs his drum, then you bang yours. Can you and your child continue taking turns to make a sequence of sounds?

- Take turns using crayons to build up a pattern. Another idea would be to take turns colouring parts of a simple picture.

- Have a puppet each. Take turns making your puppet say something, such as "Boo!", "Hello" or "Bye!"

- Use inset boards or jigsaws and take turns to fit the pieces.

6

Stage (2) 3 – 5 YEARS

At this stage children with a Semantic–Pragmatic Disorder may appear to be developing their expressive language skills very quickly. A great deal of the speech produced may be phrases that have been memorized. When the child echoes, he may be doing this to remember what he has heard. Unfortunately, the child may remember these phrases without fully understanding them. He may also say phrases but not use them to communicate.

Therapy at this stage, therefore, addresses the child's ability to understand and then build phrases, using grammatical elements. In addition, it will be helpful in developing the ways in which the child uses language to interact with others.

Giving and Listening to Instructions

Can the child take both the speaker and listener roles in the following activities? This is a useful way of showing the child how his speech can work for him and create change in his environment.

- Use a doll, brush, towel, bed and so on. First you give instructions to your child, for example, "Brush teddy", "Dry dolly", then your child directs you. Keep phrases short, stressing key words. **Handout 9** can be used to help the child formulate the instructions.

- With reuseable sticker games, let the child choose something (for example, a cat), then say, "Put it ... *in the tree*". Then you choose something and the child tells you what to do. Use **Handouts 10–12** in a similar way.

- Decide on an object to draw. Can the child tell you how to draw it? Do not draw any parts your child has not detailed. For example, if he says "legs" do not draw the feet until directed.

- Play 'Simon says' games. You give the instructions initially: for example, "Everyone ... walk/jump/sit." Then reverse roles. **Handout 13** can also be used.

- Have a line drawing each (**Handout 14 & 15**), then set up a screen between you and the child. First you give instructions: "Colour teddy's T-shirt blue ... the spade yellow..."and so on. Then, with the other picture, he directs you.

- Encourage the child to use the words 'Stop' and 'Go' to influence an activity, for example when you are both running or walking along outside or playing with push-along toys.

- Use snap cards or similar. Place one card on the table in front of the child and then start slowly to place the other cards from the pack alongside the child's card. Encourage him to shout "Stop!" when he sees a matching card.

Requesting and Listening to Requests

It may be useful to teach specific phrases to help in social situations. This will also show the child how language can be useful to him.

- Play shopping games. First you model the requests. With a very young child, or if you are aiming to raise his awareness of the basic elements of phrases, encourage key word requests: for example, "Apple, please". With older children, a useful structure would be "Can/may I have an apple, please?" **Handout 16** can be used as cue cards.

- During lotto games (for instance **Handouts 17 & 18**), or with inset puzzles, encourage requests, as in the previous example.

- When out shopping, can the child follow requests and can he choose items by making requests to you?

- Encourage the child to take an active part in dressing and undressing. For instance, can he say, "Jumper off", "Boots, please" and so on?

- Encourage the child to use the words 'more' and 'again' to request a repetition or continuation of an activity. For example, at the park, can he say, "Again" for another push on the swing?

Getting Someone's Attention

Many children do not realize that speech can work for them to gain attention. It may be of benefit to teach this skill to the child, so for instance, he can shout out or ask for help.

- Get an adult to go to the other end of the room. The child is given a useful phrase, for instance, 'Mrs Smith' or 'Come here'. Tell your child to shout this phrase to the adult (who is pretending to be doing something else). As soon as he shouts, the adult runs up and says "Yes?" or "Hello!" or whatever seems appropriate. Perhaps for extra motivation the adult could give the child a toy.

- During games, can the child indicate when it is his turn by saying, "My go!"? Work towards the child doing this unprompted.

- Roll a ball across the floor to each other. Just before you roll the ball, call out the child's name to get his attention. Can he call out your name before he rolls the ball to you?

- In a group ball game, children take turns to shout, "Me!" in order to get the ball.

Asking Questions and Answering

Children often like to ask questions to find out about their environment and make sense of people and situations.

● Take turns using picture books. First you ask, "Where is the cat?" and the child points. Then your child asks you, "Where is the dog?" and you point. You could use lotto cards (**Handouts 17 &18**) for this.

● Play a hiding game with a small toy and four cups. Ask the child, "Is it under there?", then have a look. If it isn't, try again. If you still haven't found the toy ask, "Where is it?" When the toy is found, swap roles with the child.

● Use pictures of scenes from a book (Usbourne's *First 100* **and** *1000 words* may be useful). You say, "Who is running?" and your child points. Then swap your roles.

● Have a selection of toys or pictures for your child to collect in a bag. Pick up two items and say to your child, "Which one do you want … the cow or the pig?" He answers, for example, "The pig, please." Go on like this for five or six choices. Then see if your child can ask you, "Which (do) you want … cow or … pig?".

● Put real food on a tray. Pretend to be a waiter and ask the child what he would like. Give alternatives if necessary, such as "Biscuit or apple?" When the child has 'made his order', swap roles.

● Put a toy or other object in a bag without the child seeing it. As the child feels in the bag, ask him, "What's that?" Give alternatives as prompts, if necessary. Go on like this with several different objects, then swap roles.

Giving Information

Although your child may appear to be telling you things, he may just be speaking rather than actually conversing.

● Use sound lotto tapes. First you tell the child about each sound by saying, for instance, "It's a duck!" Then take turns telling each other about the sounds.

● Use objects or photos. Take turns telling each other about them. Choose only one particular aspect to describe, such as function, colour or size. On another occasion choose a different aspect.

● Have a selection of objects and a bag. The child puts one object in the bag and you try to identify it by feel. After you have made one or two incorrect 'guesses', the child has to tell you what the object is. Then swap roles.

● Use a picture lotto game (see **Handouts 17 & 18**). The adult has the first go and selects a card, but doesn't let the child see it. Inform the child what is on the card; he then has to find the corresponding picture on the game board(s). Then it is his turn to tell you about a card.

- Use **Handout 19** and a dice. Cut the flaps (broken lines) and place pictures under them (try family photographs, object pictures and so on). Take turns rolling the dice, lifting the flaps and saying what has been 'found'.

- Whisper a word or a simple sentence to the child. Can he pass this on accurately to another person, who then repeats the message out loud?

Saying 'Yes' and 'No'
It may be useful for the child to learn to use 'yes' and 'no' appropriately, especially if he finds it hard to use appropriate non-verbal skills (for instance, facial expressions and tone of voice).

- Show the child how to use 'yes' and 'no' at mealtimes. For example, ask, "Do you want cheese?" Prompt either 'yes' or 'no' as appropriate.

- Sort some washing. Encourage the child to say 'yes' or 'no' in answer to, "Is this your/Peter's shirt?", for example.

Using Grammatical Elements
It may be useful to focus on specific grammatical elements and phrase structures and so on, so that the child is able to build his own phrases rather than just using memorized 'chunks' of language. A few basic ideas are given below.

- *Nouns*. Can the child name object pictures or photos using a single word? If the child does use a memorized phrase, repeat the relevant noun back to him. For instance, is he says, "Fireman Sam has a yellow hat", you say, "Mmm … a *hat*."

- *Verbs*. Find pictures of activities, such as, sitting or standing. See if your child can say one word to describe the picture: for example, "Sitting", not "Daddy sits on a blue chair."

- *Adjectives*. Use object pictures. Stress descriptive words in relation to the pictures: for example, 'blue', 'plastic', 'bouncy'. Go through simple object books saying, "It's *long*" (a snake), "It's *fluffy*" (a teddy) and so on.

- *Prepositions*. Have some small toys and two boxes, one upturned. Can the child say "On", "In", "Under" to tell you where to put the toys? You may have to model this first to stress the preposition.

- Use **Handouts 20–23** to make a book. Each page gives the opportunity to practise one of the above elements.

6

Stage ③ 6 – 8 YEARS

It is hoped that the child will have developed or been taught more appropriate ways of communicating with an adult at the previous stage. He must now learn to use these skills to interact more effectively with other children. Therefore it is beneficial to present activities within a small group setting, initially with one other child and then building up to a larger group. Many of the activities detailed in Stage 2 can be adapted so that the child participates in the activities with other children, rather than just with an adult. Children may find it much harder to use their developing communication skills with peers, so the adult may still need to take a leading role in the activities at Stage 3.

The track games that are included in this section can be adapted and tailored to the children and any spaces on the game sheets can be used to include extra words or categories.

Interpreting Verbal and Non-Verbal Communication

Communication relies on more than words. These activities will make the child pay attention to people's tone of voice, facial expression and body language as well as listening to their speech.

- Take turns speaking in a group. In each round a different type of information is given (for instance, favourite food, addresses). After two or three rounds the adult questions the children to find out what has been remembered: for example, "John … who liked apple pie?"

- Similarly, each child gives 'news' about their activities at the weekend or on the previous night. At the end of the round the adult asks, "James, what did John do?"

- Use sequence cards. In pairs, children discuss what is happening in the pictures. They decide the roles they are going to play, then act out the sequence for the rest of the group. The audience then say what they thought the sequence was about.

- Have each child act out different scenarios. For instance, "You are opening a present", "You feel poorly" and so on. Can the other children guess what is happening? This activity can be carried out in two other ways: (a) Without speech to encourage interpretation of non-verbal cues, (b) with the children acting out the scene behind a screen, to encourage interpretation of the language only.

- The group members form a circle and one person (an adult initially) is blindfolded. An object is passed around the group and the blindfolded person shouts, "Stop!" The person left holding the object shouts, "I've got it" and the blindfolded person says, "That's Stephen." Then take the blindfold off to check. Then children in the group volunteer to be 'it' and be blindfolded.

● Have cards (**Handout 24**) with pictures/words for feelings. In turn each child is given a short phrase (either verbally or written down depending on the needs and ability of the group). They then have to say this phrase in the 'way' specified on the card (bored, happy, sad and so on). The other children guess the feeling from the tone of voice and/or facial expression.

● Write different emotions/feelings on cards or use **Handout 24**. Children in turn try to act out the emotion shown, using facial expression and/or body language, for the others to interpret and guess.

Awareness of Conversational Rules

The child may not know how to participate in a conversation in the usual way. These skills may have to be specifically taught.

● Make a note on cards of the most usual mistakes each child makes when conversing. For example: 'Talks too fast', 'Talks at the same time as others', 'Says too much' 'Keeps changing the subject', and so on. Use these as cue cards. First two adults act out a conversation. Tell the children which adult is going to make the mistake. Can they spot the mistake? Then discuss with them how to correct these: for example, how to listen or take turns.

● From the above, draw up a chart of 'Things to remember when talking' and perhaps put this up on the wall where it can be easily referred to. Make the children aware of this, by saying for instance, "Yes, you waited for your turn to speak; well done" or "Oh dear, you talked too fast, so I couldn't understand you" and so on. *Always explain why and how the children should stick to these rules*. Don't forget, it doesn't 'go without saying'.

● Use **Handout 25**. Two adults each pick a card describing a conversational error. They then act out a short conversation, displaying these errors, in front of the group. Members of the group have to guess what was on the cards. At a later stage the children could take the adult role.

Using Relevant Language

These activities will help develop the child's awareness of the need to say pertinent things. They will also help him practise this skill.

● Have two sets of objects and give one set to each child. Put a screen up between them. One child arranges his objects and directs the other to set his out in the same way, saying for example, "Put the pencil on the plate … the bear in the cup … and the book under the plate." Encourage the listener to ask questions to clarify the instructions. Then move the screen to check whether the two sets of objects are in similar positions. Then the children reverse roles.

- Use Handout 26 and a screen (as above). One child directs the other to colour the picture as he is doing: for example, "Colour the clown's hair red", "Colour the ball under the table green."

- Similarly, one child draws a picture and directs the others to draw the same. Simple line drawings could be used as cue cards.

- Use object pictures. One child describes a picture to the others. Encourage him to say approximately four relevant things. Can the others then guess what the picture is?

- Use object pictures or objects and put them in a bag. Each child takes a turn picking up a cue card (**Handout 27**) and asking about the object. Once all the cards have been used, can the group guess what the object is?

- Use a doll's house or a toy farm. One child closes his eyes (or leaves the room) while the others hide a small counter. Then he re-enters the room (or opens his eyes) and asks questions such as "Is it under the table?" until he locates the object.

- Choose an object. One child goes out of the room and the others hide it. When the child returns the others direct him to it, *without pointing*.

- Use a picture of a washing line (**Handout 28**) and two sets of the clothes pictures (**Handout 29**). Cut one set of clothes for the line and use the others as cue cards. One child has the washing line and the other children give instructions, using the cards as cues: for example, "Hang up a long spotty sock."

- Pass an object round the group. Each person says something different about it, for example, "It's blue", "It's got a handle". Encourage the children to give information that is both relevant and succinct.

- Give the children a scene to colour (**Handout 30**), with one person giving instructions about what to colour. If anyone gives inadequate instructions, such as "Colour it blue", the others should be encouraged to ask for more information.

Inferential Skills

Your child may have developed a relatively good ability to understand at a concrete level, but may find it harder to 'read between the lines'. These activities will encourage him to infer.

- Think of a selection of different animal names, for example 'Prancer' or 'Goldie'. Can the children decide who they may belong to and discuss why? Alternatively different nick-names could be discussed (this could lead to a discussion regarding politeness and people's feelings).

- Use **Handout 31**. Cut out the speech bubbles and put them face down in a pile. Each child in turn picks one up and decides who and where the speaker might be . For example, for, "How much is it to London?" a child might decide it is a man at the station.

- Give each child paper and a pencil to draw different sorts of people, animals or monsters. Give suggestions for each one. For example, "Draw someone who is good at hearing/listening (might have big ears)", "Draw an animal that can smell things well (might have a big nose)."

- Use **Handout 32** giving true and false statements, such as "I have 27 brothers", "I have two sisters", "I am 65 years old" or "I am 25 years old". Mix these up. Can the children decide which could be true and which could not? Make the differences more or less obvious to suit the skills of the group.

- Use sequencing pictures. One child has to turn away while the pictures are put in a sequence and one picture is covered up. The child who is 'it' then turns back and tries to work out what was happening in the picture that is covered. Use three-picture sequences for younger children, working up to longer ones for the older children.

Sequencing & Temporal Language Skills

By this stage the child will have developed an understanding of concrete concepts. More abstract ideas such as 'time' may continue to cause difficulties.

- Use object pictures and give one to each child. The first child starts a story, including in it the object on his picture. Each child then adds to the story, including the items on their cards. To make this activity more difficult, give the story a theme such as 'A scary story' or 'A happy story'.

- Choose a sequential task, such as making egg sandwiches, planting seeds or doing a craft activity. Can the group think of all the steps needed to complete the task? Perhaps draw or write the steps on cards and use them to identify gaps or errors in the sequence. The group then carry out the task, using the cards as a reference.

- Use sequencing cards such as those developed above. Ask questions using time concept words ('first', 'next', 'last' and 'then', 'before', 'after'): for instance, "What did we do first?", "What did we do before …?"

- Use diaries or make timetables (**Handout 33**) for the school day. Use them as suggested in the previous activity.

- Play "I went to market and I bought … ", where each child recalls in sequence what has been said before and adds an item. You can vary this by changing the scene: for instance, "I went on holiday to Spain and

6

I packed ... "; or by choosing a category of items such as toys, fruit or zoo animals. A narrow category (vegetables) would be more difficult than a wide one (food).

● One child is 'it' and gives another child (or other children in turn) sequences of instructions. For instance, "Point to the floor, then the table, then the window." Or "Get me a book, a pencil and a pair of scissors, please." Then another child takes his turn to give the instruction. Cue cards (**Handout 34**), could also be used. To make this harder, the objects should be set down in the correct sequence, from left to right.

Grammatical Skills

The child may continue to have difficulties formulating specific phrases, as a great deal of his speech may be composed of memorized 'chunks' of language. Further work on the grammatical elements of language may therefore help him create new phrases.

● To practise the past tense, get the children to close their eyes and listen as the adult does something, such as stamping her feet. The children then open their eyes and say what happened: "You stamped your feet!", "You tapped the table", and so on.

● To practise the future tense, act as if you are just about to do something, such as clap your hands, open a door, and so on. Ask "what will I do?" The children then say, for example, "You are going to kick that ball."

● Use the adjective track game (**Handout 35**) and some counters. When a child lands on an adjective picture (such as 'round') he has to think of something that word describes and put it into a phrase: for instance, 'a round wheel'.

● During group activities encourage the use of personal pronouns (I, me, mine, yours). For example, during lotto games children can shout out, "It's mine!" When giving out toys or pictures ask, "Who wants this?" and wait for the response, "Me!" Also encourage the use of "My turn!" in turn-taking games.

● Use category pictures (**Handout 36**) and work in pairs. Each person collects pictures of one category. One of the pair takes the pictures from a pile saying, "That's mine", "It's yours" and so on. After several turns the other person is the speaker.

Vocabulary Skills

The child may have learnt many words, especially in relation to his interests. Other words may have been acquired within memorized phrases. However, there may not be an underlying understanding of the concepts that help vocabularies develop normally.

- Use **Handout 36** and cut out the pictures. Each child collects one category (for instance, Transport). One person (initially the adult) calls out "Lorry!" or whatever is on the picture. Everyone listens and the person collecting the appropriate category shouts out "Mine!"

- A harder activity would be as above, but using **Handout 37**, where the categories are more similar.

- The adult decides on a category. Each child has to think of an item from that category.

- Use **Handout 38**, a dice game for two or more players, to think of items within categories.

- Use **Handouts 39–42**. Can the child decide which is the odd one out and say why? The sheets increase in difficulty.

- Use **Handout 43**. Cut out the pictures. Can your child sort them into pairs and explain the connection to you? You can also use the pictures to play a memory game: with pictures face down on the table, take turns to turn two over; you win them if they are a pair.

- A much harder game, using the same, or any pictures of objects, would be to select two cards at random and try to think of a link between them. If you can think of one then you win the cards.

- Use the opposites pictures in **Handouts 44 & 45**. Have two copies of each to make lotto cards and boards. Play as a lotto game. For a slightly harder game, the adult calls out a word and the children cover up its opposite, using counters.

- Use **Handout 46**, a dice game where the child has to think of the opposite of a given word.

6

Stage ④ 9 YEARS AND OVER

Awareness of Other People's Thoughts

Some individuals find it difficult to appreciate that what they know is not necessarily shared by others. This difficulty can be severe or quite subtle. It is bound to have an effect on that person's ability to converse using pertinent and clear information. It is also likely to affect the development of his ability to use and interpret non-verbal cues, such as facial expressions.

- Use a selection of everyday objects and a screen. One child sets out the objects as he wishes, behind a screen. Another child then tries to guess how the objects have been arranged. When this person guesses incorrectly, discuss with the children why this has happened. ("You knew, but he didn't, because he couldn't see them.")

- Play Battleships. Each person has a different grid with ships marked on it. In turn, players guess where the other's ships are located (for example, 'B4'), to get the response "Hit!" or "Miss!" A successful guess can help a player to deduce where other ships are. This game will help the child appreciate that not all knowledge is shared.

- Role-play activities encourage children to put themselves in somebody else's shoes. Video recordings can be made to promote discussion afterwards. For instance, "Would the lady standing in the bus queue really have talked about trains?"

- Use **Handout 47** or photos and some catalogues. Can the children choose appropriate presents from the catalogues for the people described? Discuss with the group why the people may like or need the things chosen. If using photos, start with more familiar people such as family members.

- For older children, use estate agents' pamphlets describing houses and give the children short descriptions of people or families (**Handout 48**). Can they work out which houses would be suitable for which people?

- Get the children to make up suitable food shopping lists for the people in **Handout 49**. (Each child in the group could be allocated a person for whom to shop.) Then they should read out their list to the rest of the group for discussion.

- As above, but this time the children have to choose clothes for different occasions for the people in **Handout 47**. You can use catalogues for ideas.

- One person is 'it' and leaves the room. The others then place an object somewhere in the room (a sticky note pad page is good to use for this). The person waiting outside then comes back in with his eyes closed (or is blindfolded if he agrees to this) and the others guide him *verbally* to the object. They can either take turns giving instructons or direct him as a group.

Finding Out About Others

Even at this age the child may be quite egocentric and only remember what interests and benefits him.

- Use a track game (**Handout 50**). When the children land on a star, they must ask another child a question to find out something about them. Another game would be to play as above, but using cards (**Handout 51**) which specify the question type.

- Choose a category such as favourite foods or other likes/dislikes. In turn, members of the group give their information. Go round the group twice. The adult then asks, "Peter, who didn't like cabbage?", "Ben, who liked carrots?" and so on.

- Use the questionnaire sheets (**Handout 52**). Initially, children use the questionnaires to 'interview' other group members and report back what they have found out. This could be extended by the children interviewing others outside the group setting and reporting back to the group at a later date.

Working Together as a Group

The child may operate as an individual and not see himself as part of a larger group. These activities will force him to work with others.

- Tell the children to organize themselves into a line (working from left to right) starting with the tallest person and going down to the shortest. Try not to help!

- As above, but appoint one person to *direct* the others.

- A much more difficult game would be as in the previous two, but with the children having to ask each other for information first: for example, arranging themselves from youngest to oldest, or according to the distance they live from school.

- Go around the group, making up a phrase or sentence by adding a word each time. For example, the first person says "I", the second says, "I went", the third, "I went to" and so on.

- Write the words of a sentence on individual cards. (If you have a group of six, then choose a six-word sentence, and so on.) Give each group member a card to hold up. Then let the group sort themselves into a line in the correct order to form the sentence. You could vary this by choosing one person to direct the others, or instructing the group to carry out the task without speaking.

- Use construction bricks. Draw on cards diagrams of from six to ten-piece constructions (whatever is appropriate to the size of the group). Place red bricks on a plate, green in a box, yellow in a bag, and so on. One person closes their eyes and the others, taking turns, then direct him in order to make the model depicted on a card.

Inferential Skills and Non-Literal Language

We do not always say what we mean, but use language in more abstract ways. The child must learn to be flexible in the way he interprets language.

- Give the children two pieces of information to draw together to make a conclusion. For example, "I am going to bake a cake … [3–4 second pause] … I like chocolate." Ask, "What flavour cake will I make?". **Handout 53** gives further examples.

- Use pictures of objects. Put five or six on the table. In turn, participants choose someone to listen, then they say one word in connection with one of the pictures: for instance, 'time' in relation to a picture of a radio (as the time is given on the radio). Encourage them to give clues which are as cryptic as possible. The other person has to make the connection and then point to the relevant card.

- Use examples of metaphor, proverbs and so on (often to be found in dictionaries). Talk about the implied meaning of these phrases and how they do not mean what they actually say.

- Watch television programmes, looking out for examples of non-literal language. The group could also do this for homework.

Language and Vocabulary Styles

Language is used in a variety of ways to make it appropriate to the given situation. Selecting the tone of voice and/or speech 'code' can make or break a communicative attempt.

- Use **Handouts 54–56**, counters and a dice. Cut **Handout 54** into strips and **Handout 55** into cards. Participants throw the dice and move round the track (**Handout 56**). When someone lands on a speech bubble, they pick up a card and a strip and then decide if they go together. For instance, "Oi, shift up!"— to a headteacher?

- Get the group participants to think of different ways we use language: for example, interviewing, making a speech, giving directions, conversation, reading aloud, asking questions in class, and so on. The group then practise these different ways of using language in role-play activities. Participants could, for example, act out making a speech for the others to guess the language use or style.

- To practise appropriate tone of voice and facial expression, use any picture cards and write the following pairs on blank cards: like–dislike, puzzled–sure/confident, asking–answering, happy–sad. Each child, in turn, picks up a picture from the pack and one word pair, which he shows to the other participants. He then says the name of the item on the card (use only the single word), expressing his like or dislike of it and so on. The others then guess the emotion. Harder activities would be to have all the word pairs on show and the partipants having to guess the emotion from all the possibilities, or for the person speaking to hide his face so that the others have to guess by interpreting tone of voice only.

- Using a large sheet of paper to make notes, have a brainstorming session. Can the participants think of positive and negative words that relate to people, such as 'polite', 'nasty' or 'selfish'? Make two lists of positive and negative characteristics. Can the children decide which list their word goes in? When a selection of words has been noted, can the chidren, in turn, act out these characteristics?

- Use any dice game and the synonym cards (**Handout 57**). After each move, the player picks up a card and has to think of a synonym, such as 'freezing' for 'cold'. If the player cannot think of one, he must go back one space. For older children, or to get more examples, use a thesaurus.

- To develop the child's flexibility in use of vocabulary, use words such as those listed below. Each of these words has at least two different meanings (homographs). Can the group members think of sentences to show these different meanings?

mark	cross	jam	ring
drive	felt	left	flat
bay	duck	lie	hard
jack	bat	lean	watch
light	navy	round	post

- Think of several different professions and write them on cards. In pairs, the participants choose a card, then one interviews the other for that job. Discuss afterwards the relevance of their questions and responses.

- Use telephone extensions to practise telephone skills. Perhaps give one person a few short messages or phrases for the other to listen to and remember.

- As above, use telephone extensions but give the listener ten simple noun or verb pictures on cards. Give the speaker a written list of five of these words. He then goes through this list and the listener lines up the relevant cards. Then go into the listener's room with the list to check the results.

- Teach appropriate telephone skills such as using 'tags', "Mmmm", "Oh yes" and so on, and also "Hi" and "Bye". Make a note of particular difficulties the children have and work on these.

- Cut several similar pictures, such as trains or cars, from magazines. Number them on the back. The participants record descriptions of the pictures (in order) on a tape when the adult is out of the room. The pictures are then muddled up and the adult comes in and listens to the recording, identifying them: "Number two was ... that one!" Then check on the back to see if this is correct.

- Use Handout 58. Can the participants choose a card and then decide: (a) should you approach this person/these people, (b) what might you say, and (c) how would you say it (tone of voice and so on)?

Conversational Skills

Usually, we know instinctively how to join a conversation and stay involved in it. The child may have to be taught these skills.

- Think up phrases that typically start, continue or finish a conversation, for example, "Hello, how are you" or less obvious, "I haven't seen you for a while", "Well, long time no see!" Also, "Oh, by the way", "Can I just say?" or "Oh, look at the time!". Can the children decide where they might occur in a conversation and discuss why?

- Write the phrases from the activity above on blank cards. In pairs, can the children 'chat' about a given topic, for instance holidays. One child has a card with a phrase and must bring it into the conversation. Other members of the group assess whether he used the phrase at an appropriate time. An adult may need to go first (with a card/phrase) to demonstrate the task.

- As homework, the group members must watch a television programme and write down a number of conversational 'starters' or 'finishers'. Other members of the group then act out the scenario to this person's instructions. (They may need to decide on suitable programmes beforehand, as factual programmes would not necessarily include conversations.)

- To practise 'staying on topic' use pictures of everyday objects. One card is selected and the group must have a conversation that includes this or relates to it in some way. If anyone switches topic without any obvious connection being made, then stop the dialogue and discuss what has happened.

Semantic-Pragmatic
LANGUAGE DISORDER

Katherine Venkatesh

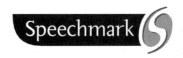

Telford Road • Bicester • Oxon OX26 4LQ • UK

Editor's Note

For the sake of clarity alone, in this pack we have used 'he' to refer to the child.

Published by
Speechmark Publishing Ltd, Telford Road, Bicester, Oxon OX26 4LQ
United Kingdom
www.speechmark.net

© Charlotte Firth & Katherine Venkatesh, 1999
First published 1999
Reprinted 2001, 2002, 2003

002-3342/Printed in the United Kingdom/1030
British Library Cataloguing in Publication Data
Firth, Charlotte,
    Photocopiable therapy handouts
    Part 3 Charlotte Firth, Katherine Venkatesh
    1. Speech disorders in children 2. Speech disorders in children – Diagnosis
    3. Speech therapy for children
    I. Title II. Venkatesh, Katherine
    618.9'2855'06

ISBN for Part 3: 0 86388 328 1
ISBN for complete set of 3 volumes: ISBN 0 86388 329 X
ISBN for Part 1: 0 86388 326 5
ISBN for Part 2: 0 86388 327 3
Previously published by Winslow Press Ltd under ISBN 0 86388 240 4 (Part 1), 0 86388 241 2 (Part 2), 0 86388 242 0 (Part 3), 0 86388 203 X (complete set)

HANDOUTS

1 ● Eye Contact

2 ● Eye Contact

3 ● Pointing

4 ● Cause & Effect

5 ● Making Choices

6 ● Symbols

7 ● Joint Activities

8 ● Turn Taking

9–15 ● Giving & Listening to Instructions

16 ● Shopping Games

17–18 ● Picture Lotto Game

19 ● Dice Game

20–23 ● Nouns, Verbs, Adjectives & Prepositions

24 ● Feelings

25 ● Conversational Errors

26 ● Colouring Pictures

27 ● Cue Cards

28 & 29 ● Washing Line & Clothes

30 ● A Scene to Colour

31 ● Speech Bubbles

32 ● True & False

33 ● School Day

34 ● Sequences

35 ● Adjective Track Game

36 & 37 ● Category Pictures

38 ● Category Dice Game

39–42 ● Odd One Out

43 ● Pairs

44 & 45 ● Opposites

46 ● Opposites Dice Game

47–49 ● People & Families

50 & 51 ● Ask a Question Games

52 ● Questionnaire

53 ● Can You Work it Out?

54–56 ● Would You Say That? Track Game

57 ● Synonyms

58 ● Social Skills Cards

1

Eye Contact

Eye contact is a very important part of communicating.

- Hold toys next to your face as you name them. For example, say, "Look ... a car."

- See if your child notices something silly (a cup, for example) balanced on your head. If not, get him to look at you and to take it off.

- Play peek-a-boo games with your child where you hide your face.

- Put stickers on your nose. Encourage your child to look at you and to pull the stickers off.

- Let your child brush your hair, wash your face, put face paints on you, and so on.

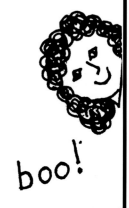

boo!

2

Eye Contact

Eye contact can be used to get people's attention.

● Use toys that can be activated, such as wind-up toys. When your child looks at the toy and then at you, activate the toy.

● Use bubbles. When your child looks at the container of bubble mixture and then at you, blow some more bubbles.

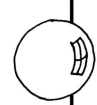

● At mealtimes have a choice of foods. Encourage your child to choose one by looking at the food and then at you.

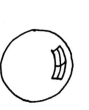
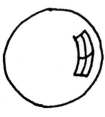

3

Pointing

Pointing helps us to communicate our wants and needs.

● Encourage your child to point to things to indicate his preferences. Do this by giving choices at mealtimes, when getting dressed, when playing with toys, and so on.

● Put a favourite toy out of your child's reach. Show your child how to point to it and give the toy to him when he does this.

● Use picture books. Encourage your child to point to the pictures for you to name. When your child makes a recognizable attempt at pointing, name the picture quickly so that he links the two things together.

● When you go out for a walk, encourage your child to point to things that he would like to investigate.

4

Cause & Effect

In order to communicate we need to understand how to make things happen.

● Choose toys that need switches to activate them, or that make sounds or movements (eg. jack-in-the-box, pop-up farm).

● Use your child's vocalizations. When he makes a sound (even if this is not purposeful) give him a toy, food, and so on. See if he starts to realize that sounds can be used to communicate with people.

● Play a game with a doll. Pretend the doll is asleep. Say "Shh ... dolly's asleep". Then model getting close to the doll and saying, "Boo!" Make the doll jump up and act frightened. Then she goes to sleep again. Can you get your child to say 'Boo!' (or any sound initially) as the trigger to wake up the doll?

● Build a tower of bricks and wait for your child to make a sound before the teddy knocks it down. You could also use this idea with toy cars going down a ramp, or with you kicking a ball.

Making Choices

Making choices gives your child a chance to communicate his ideas.

● Encourage your child to choose constantly: at mealtimes, when getting dressed, at play. Say, for example, "Do you want milk or orange?", "Shall we give dolly a drink or some dinner?" Encourage eye pointing or gestures if your child does not use words.

● In play, set up activities for teddy and dolly. Ask, for example, "Does teddy want dinner or a drink?"; "What shall dolly do now: sleep or jump?"; "Who wants the hat: teddy or dolly?"

● Use an inset puzzle. Ask your child to choose which pieces to put back in.

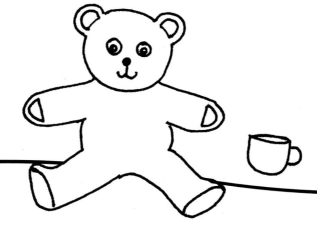

6

Symbols

Pictures, toys, drawings and sounds are all symbols for real objects.

- Play object picture matching games. Can your child match objects, first to photographs, then to coloured drawings, then to line drawings?

- Encourage pretend play. First, you and your child act out everyday situations. Then try sequences with dolls and toys (getting up, getting dressed, and so on). Finally, work towards using small doll's houses and similar toys.

- Your child may try to act out scenes from favourite books or videos and use these characters. Try to develop this into more make-believe play by bringing in other elements, such as animals, people or situations.

- Encourage your child to draw simple line drawings, such as faces or people. Talk through them as you draw together.

- Accompany play with sound effects such as 'brrm' for cars, noises for animals, and so on.

7

Joint Activities

Playing with others is one of the first steps towards communication.

● Play joint action games, such as 'Row, row, row your boat ...'

● Play finger rhymes such as, 'Round and round the garden'. Watch out for your child trying to initiate these games if he enjoys them, for example by holding out his hand.

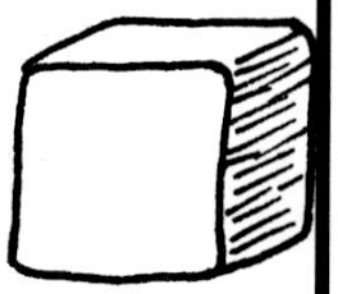

● In a group everyone has a cup. One person has small beads or bricks in theirs (or water, if you are feeling brave!). This person pours the beads or bricks into the next person's cup, who then pours them into the next, and so on. This is more difficult if you can use only one hand, as this requires more joint attention.

● Use construction toys. Join in with your child as he makes a simple model. As he becomes used to this, give more direct suggestions.

● Sit facing your child. Use cars, a ball, wheeled toys and so on to push/roll to each other. You or your child could say "Go!" to get the other person to push the toy.

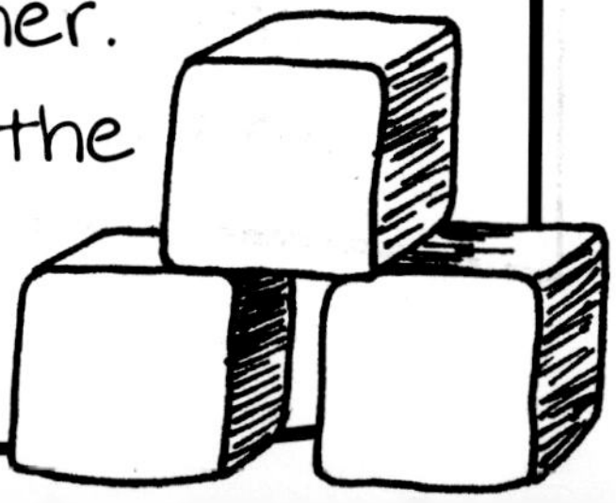

P

8

Turn taking

Turn taking is the basis of two-way interaction.

● Build a tower, taking turns to add the bricks.

● Take turns threading large beads onto a string.

● Use pairs of noisemakers (shakers, tambourines, drums). Take turns making sounds. For example, your child bangs his drum, then you bang yours. Can you and your child continue taking turns to make a sequence of sounds?

● Take turns using crayons to build up a pattern. Another idea would be to take turns colouring parts of a simple picture.

● Have a puppet each. Take turns making your puppets say something such as "Boo!", "Hello" or "Bye!"

● Use inset puzzles or jigsaws, taking turns to fit the pieces.

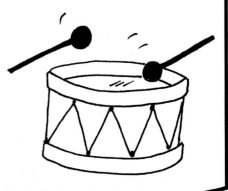

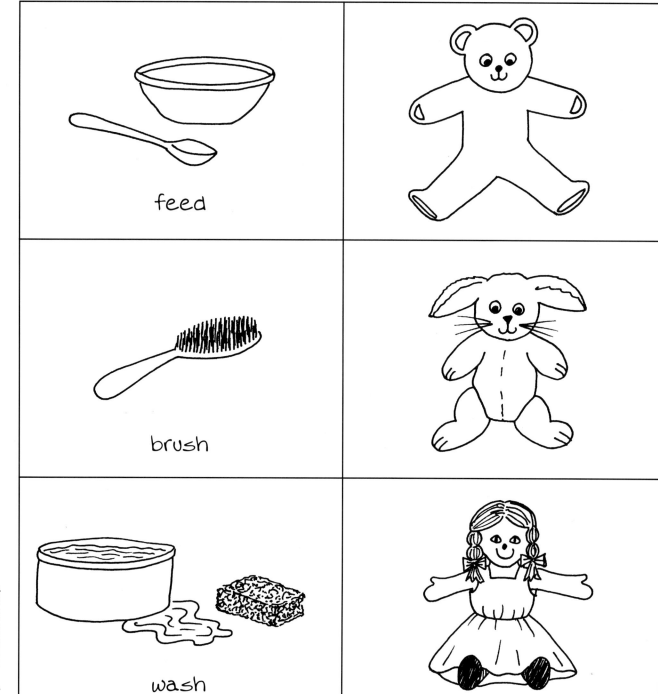

feed

brush

wash

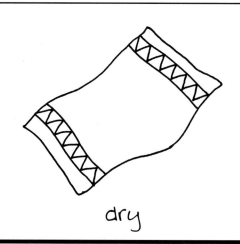

dry

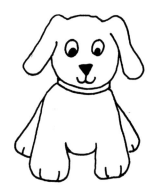

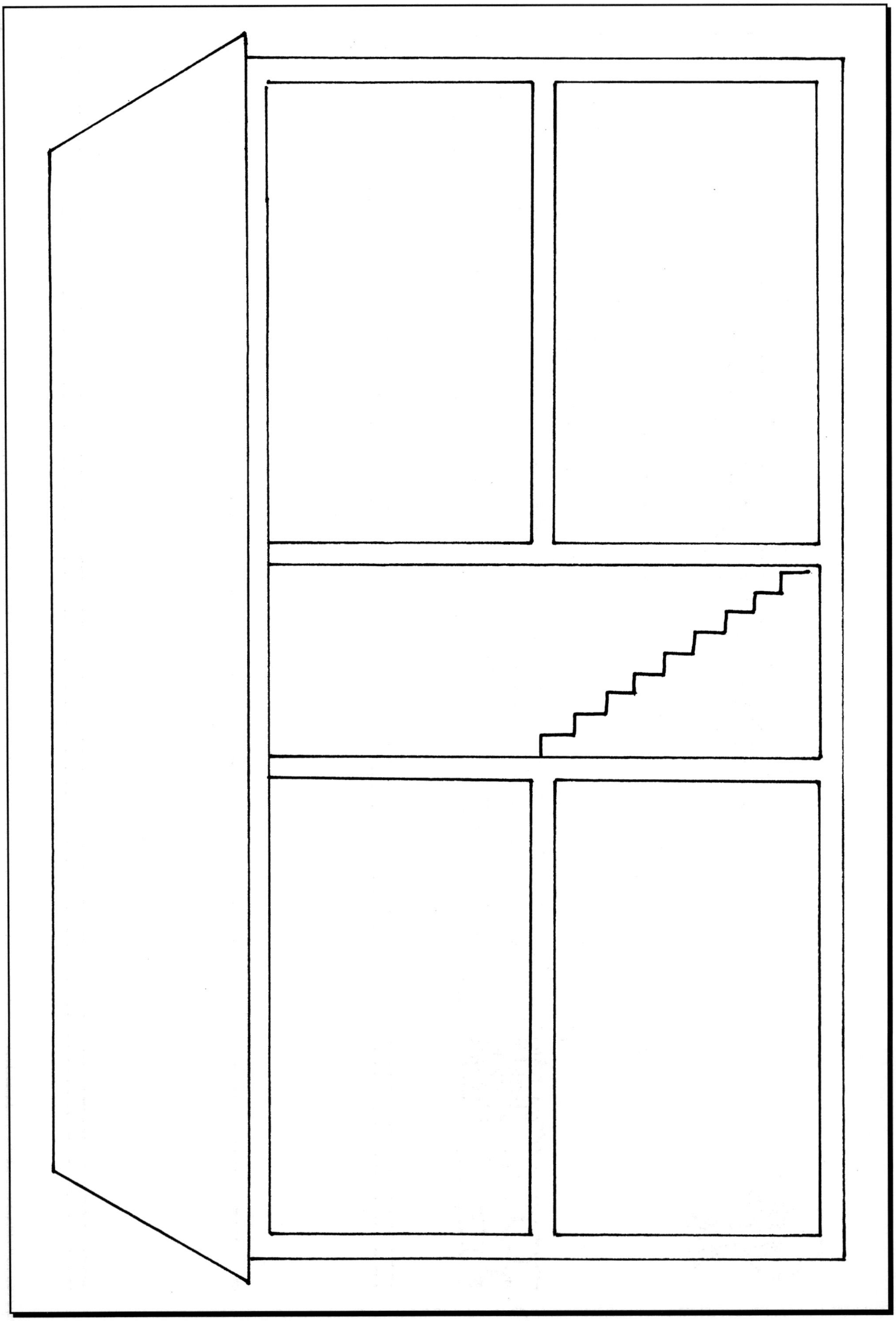

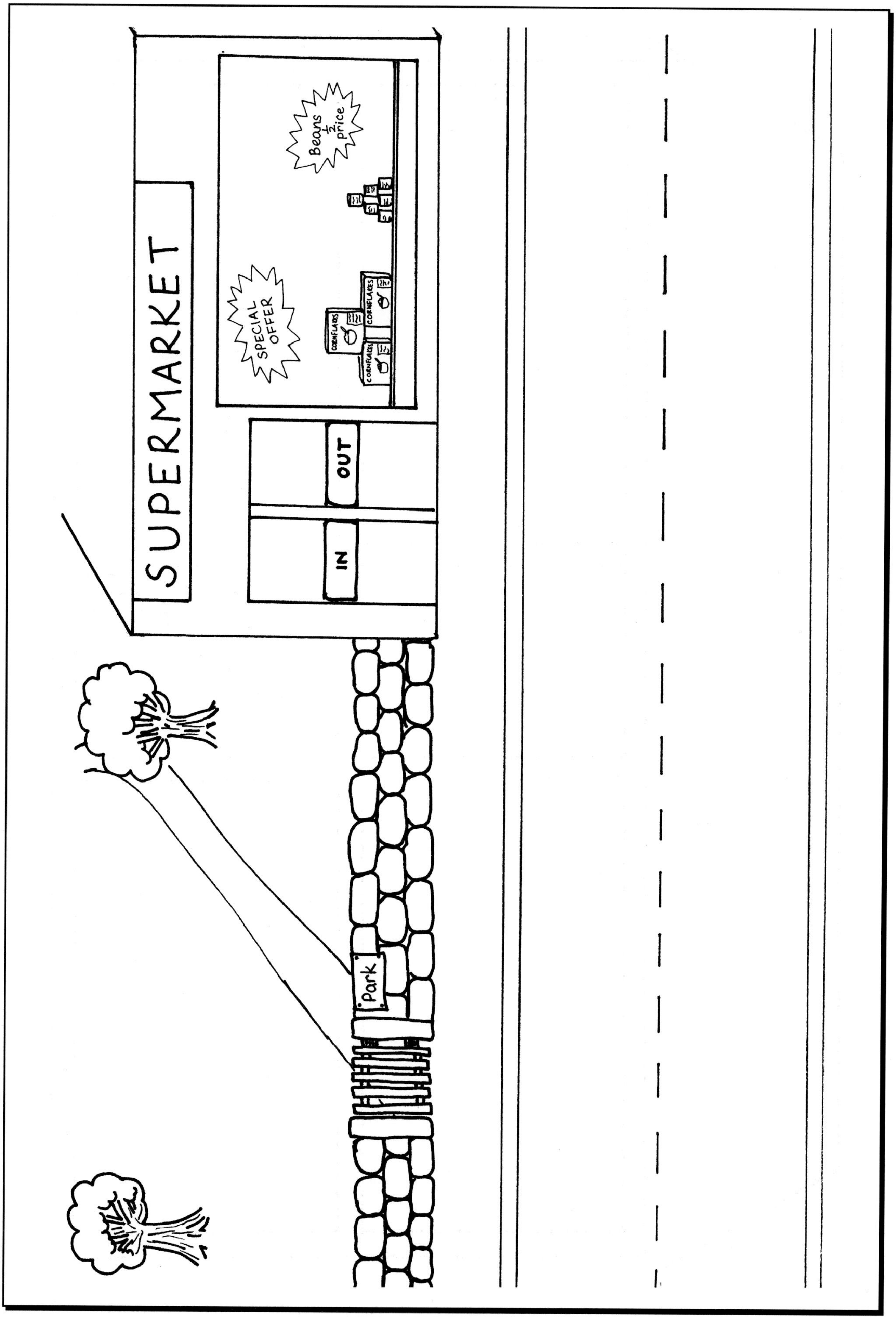

SUPERMARKET

SPECIAL OFFER

Beans ½ price

IN

OUT

CORNFLAKES

CORNFLAKES

CORNFLAKES

Park

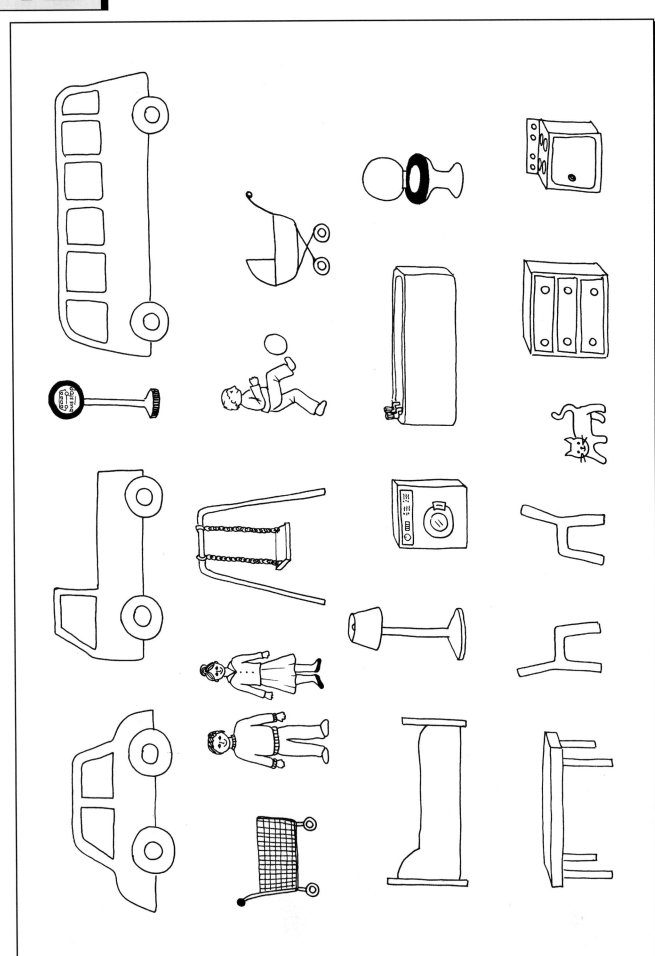

run

wave

stand

jump

sit

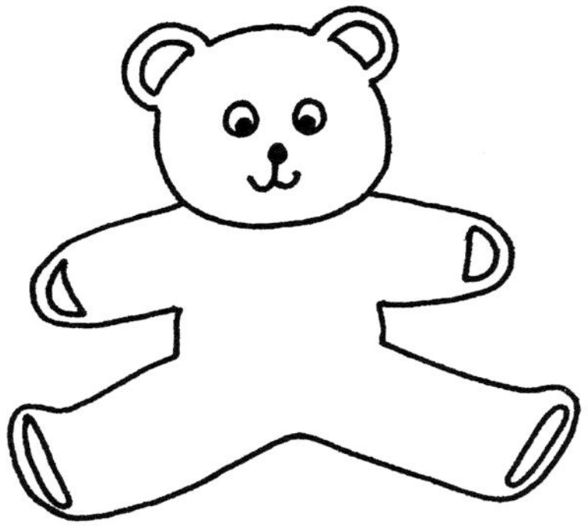

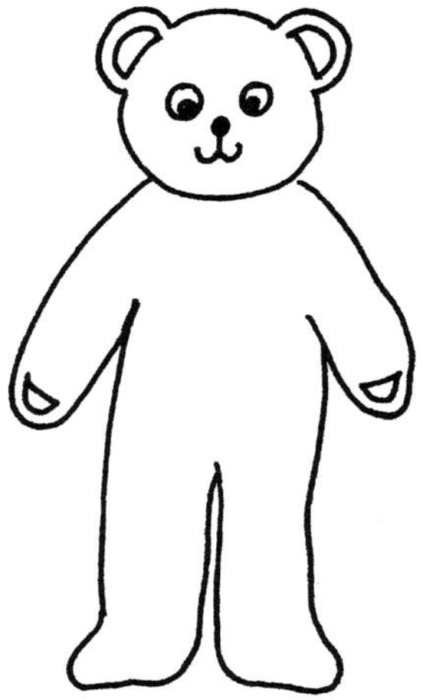

sleep

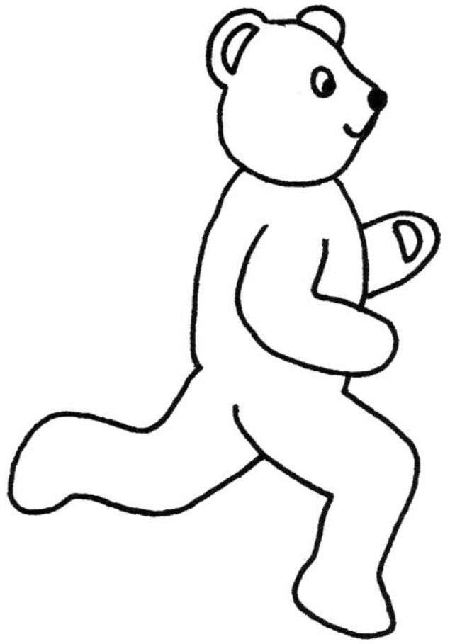

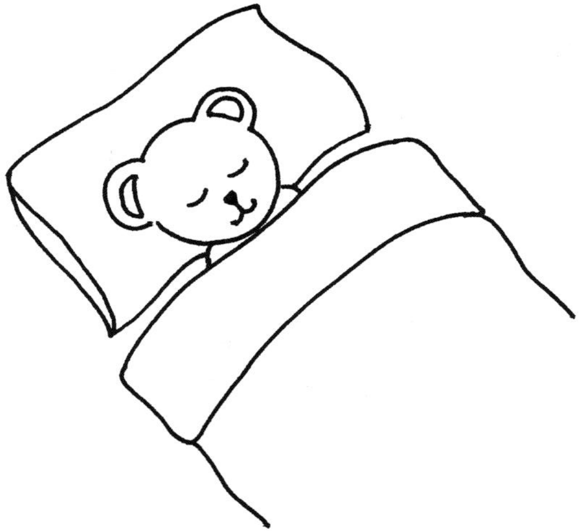

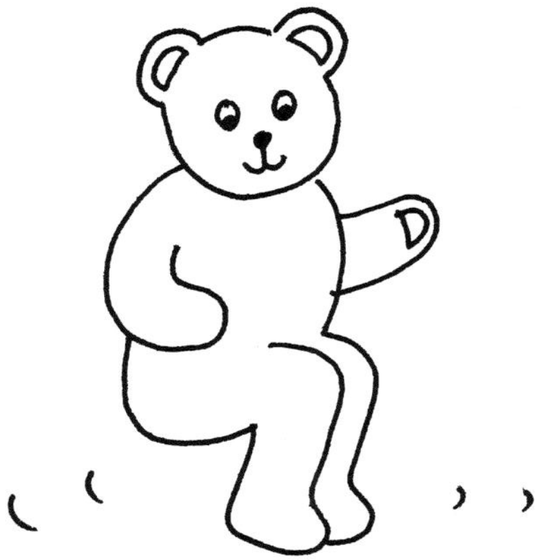

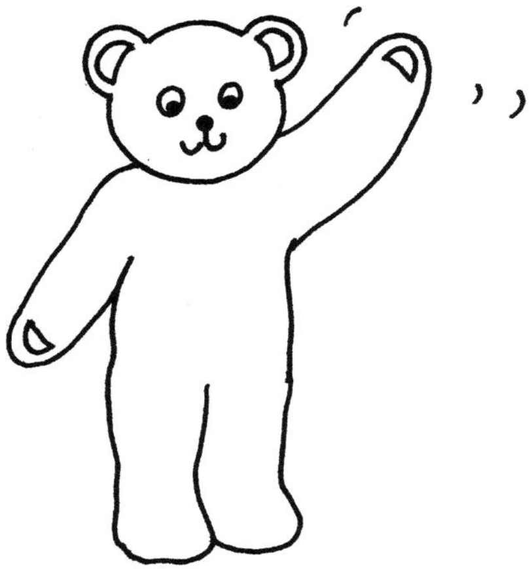

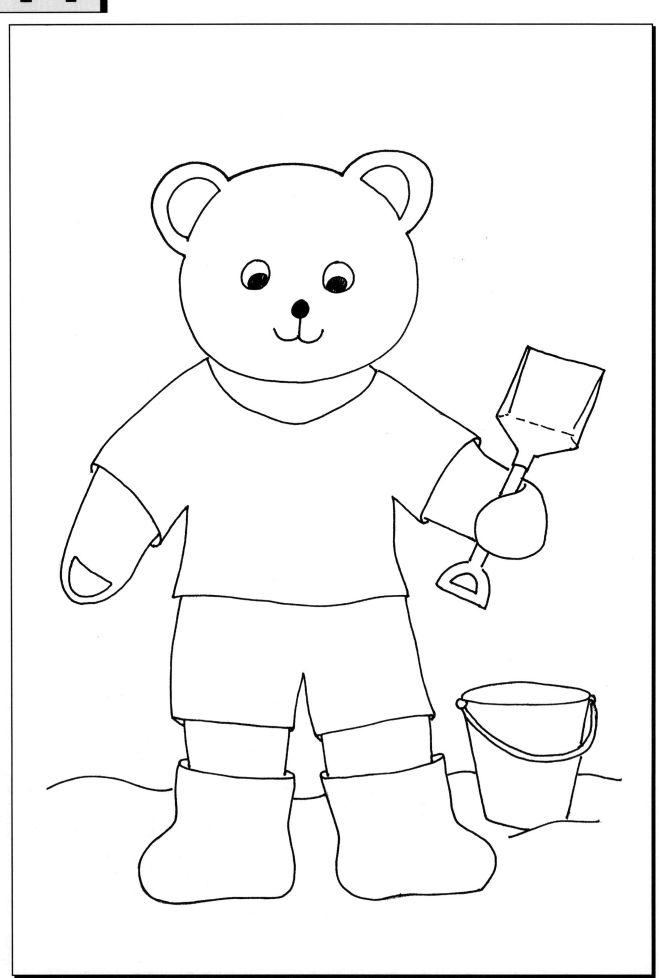

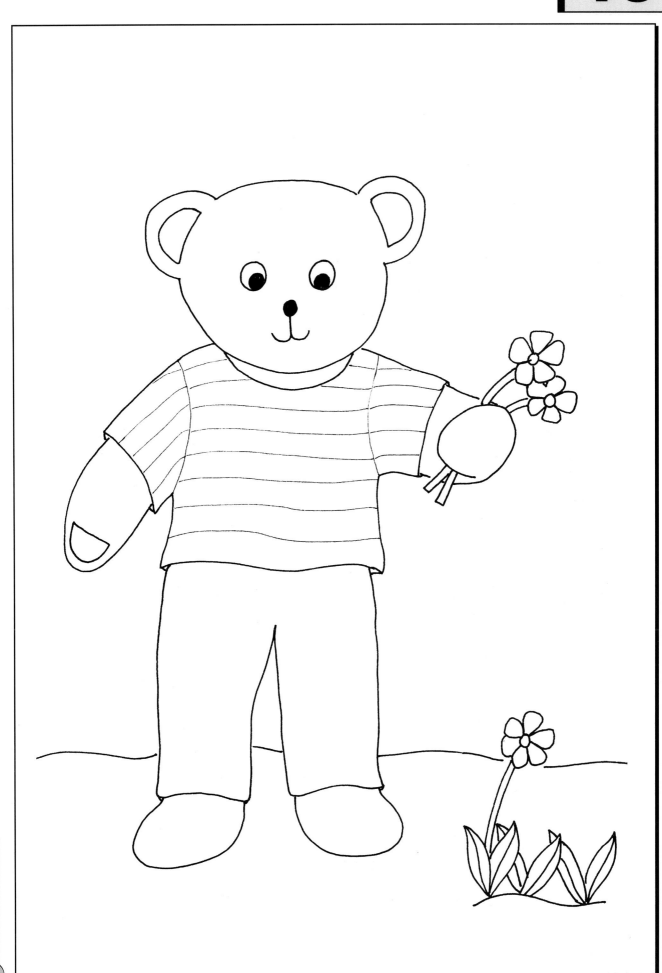

16

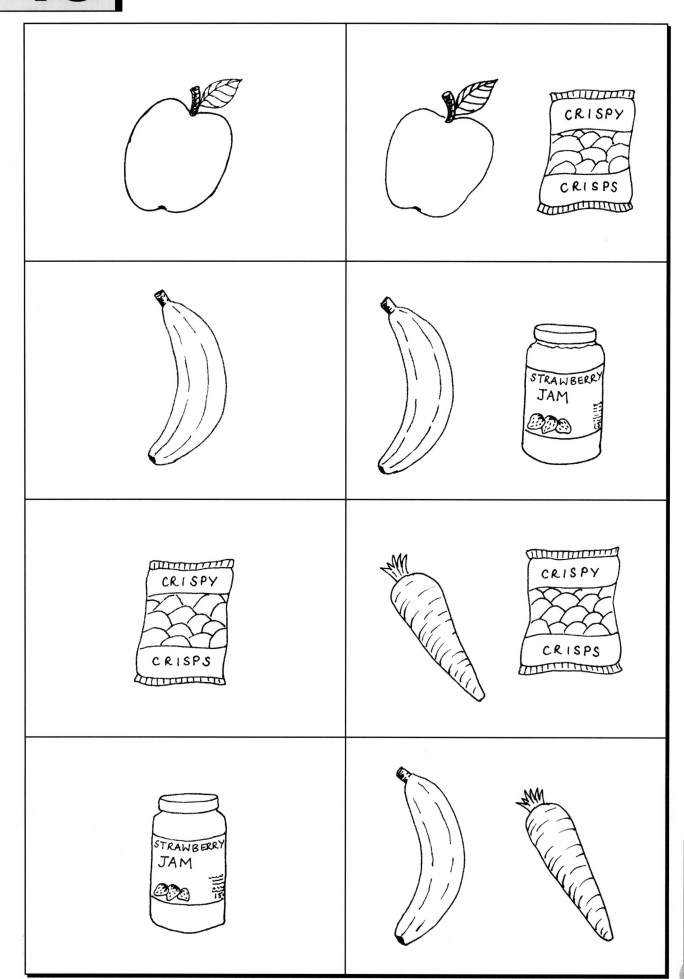

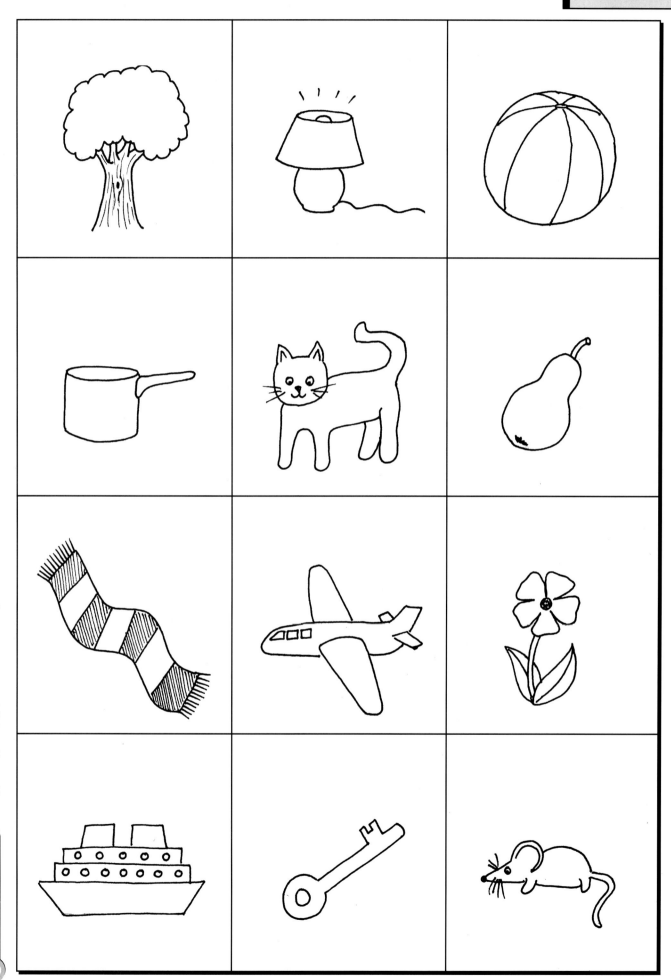

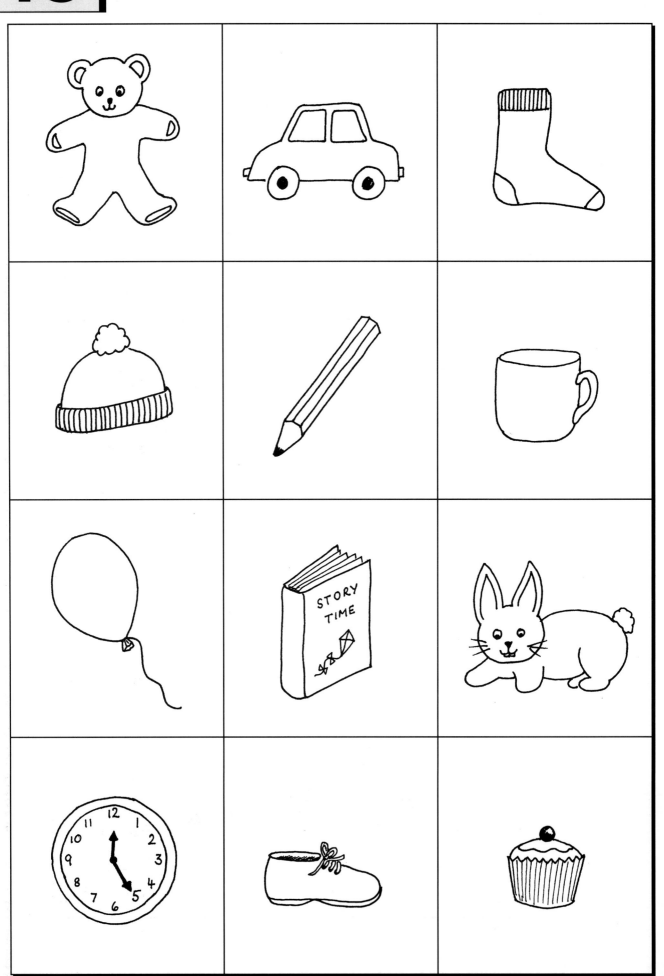

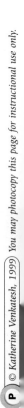

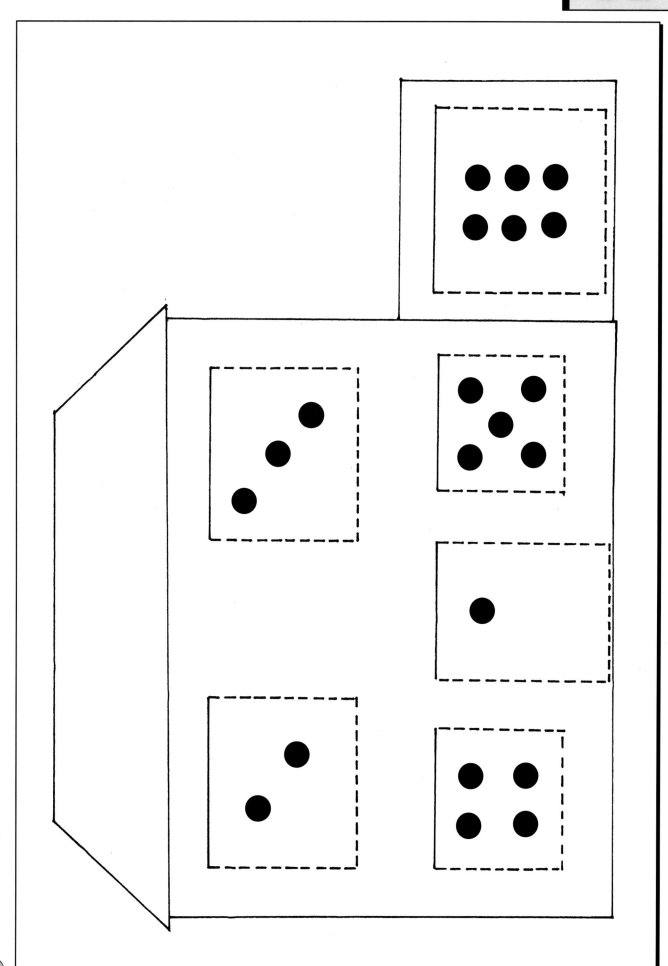

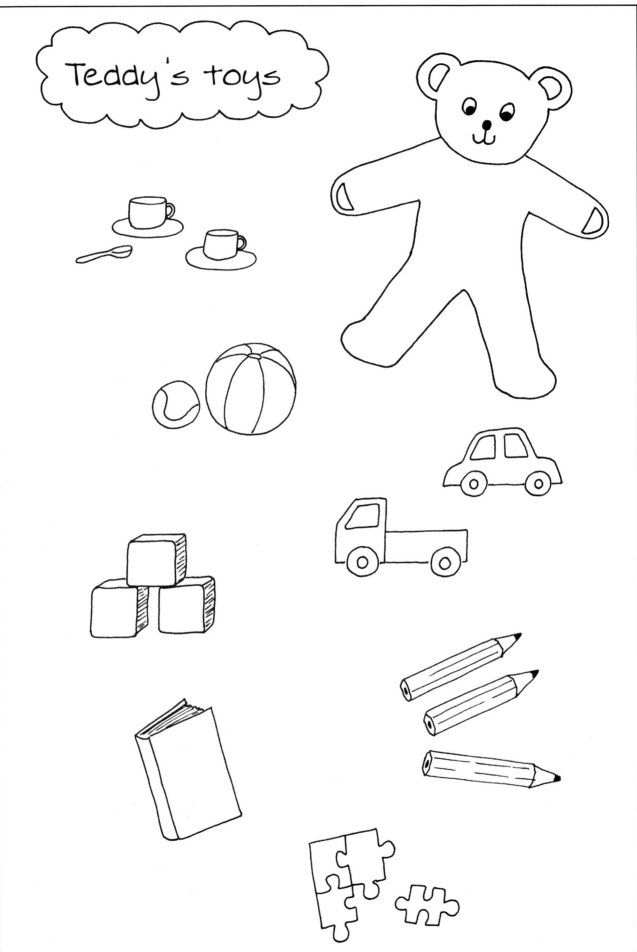

Teddy's toys

What is teddy doing?

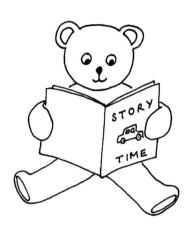

reading

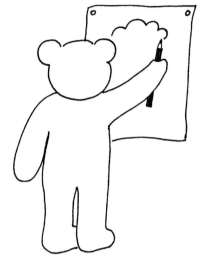

drawing

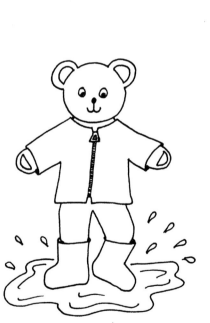

splashing

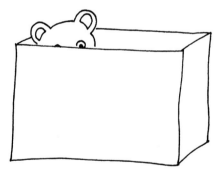

hiding

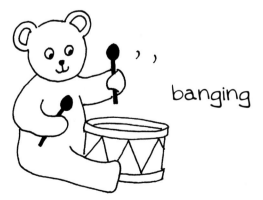

banging

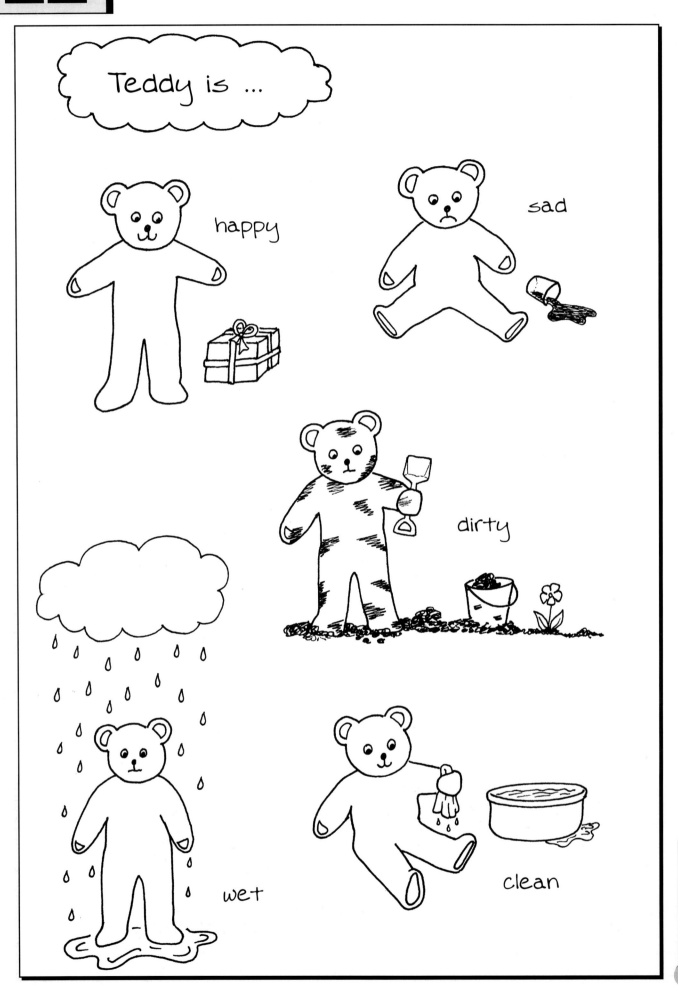

Teddy is ...

happy

sad

dirty

wet

clean

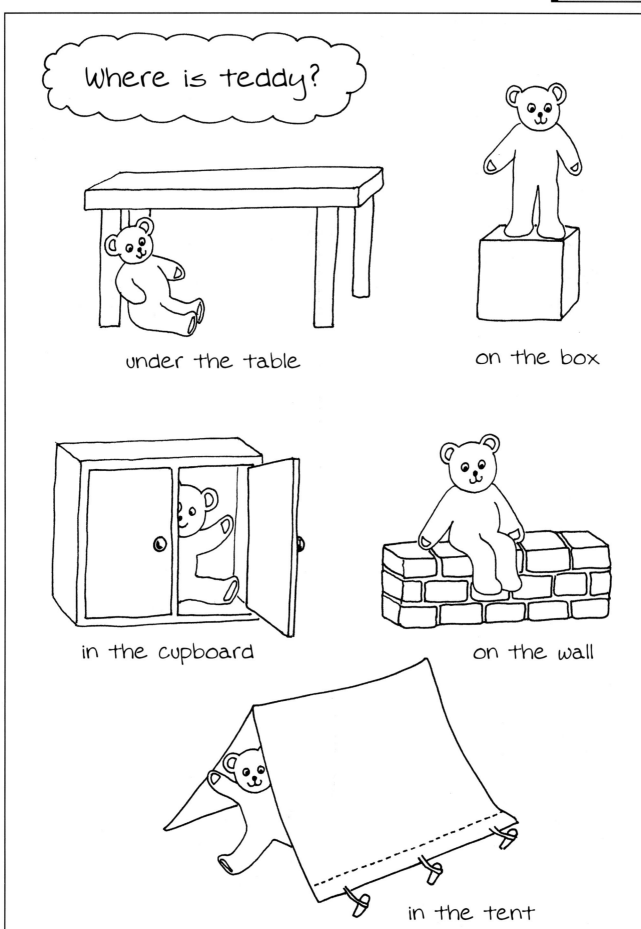

Where is teddy?

under the table

on the box

in the cupboard

on the wall

in the tent

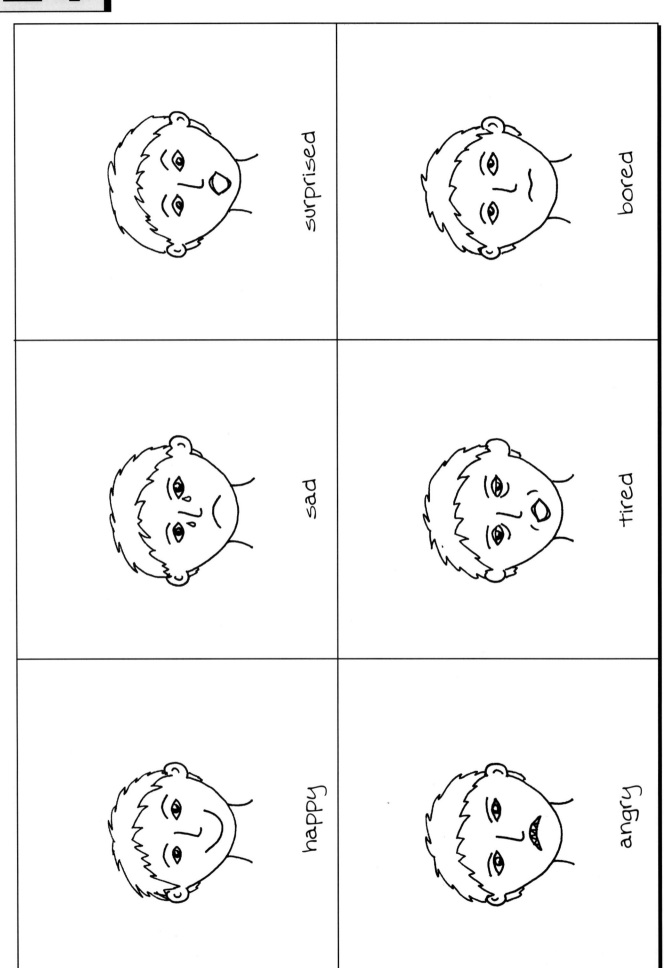

surprised

bored

sad

tired

happy

angry

Talk at the same time as the other person	Mumble quietly
Change the subject	Ask too many questions
Sit too close	Face away from the speaker
Talk with a loud voice	Fidget

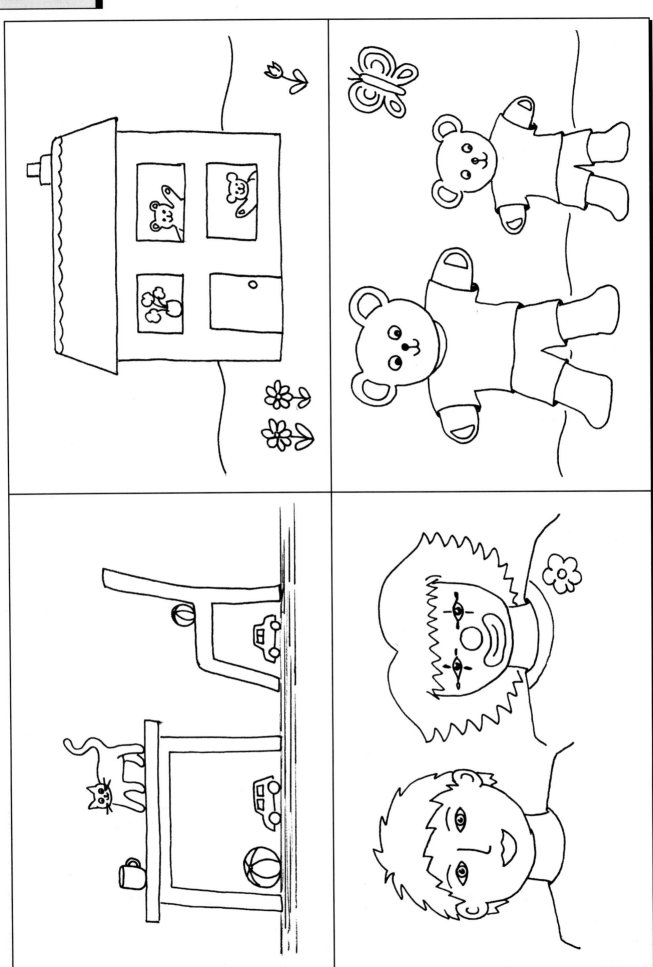

27

Colour?

Shape?

Feel?

Size?

Used for?

Made of?

Eat it?

Is it alive?

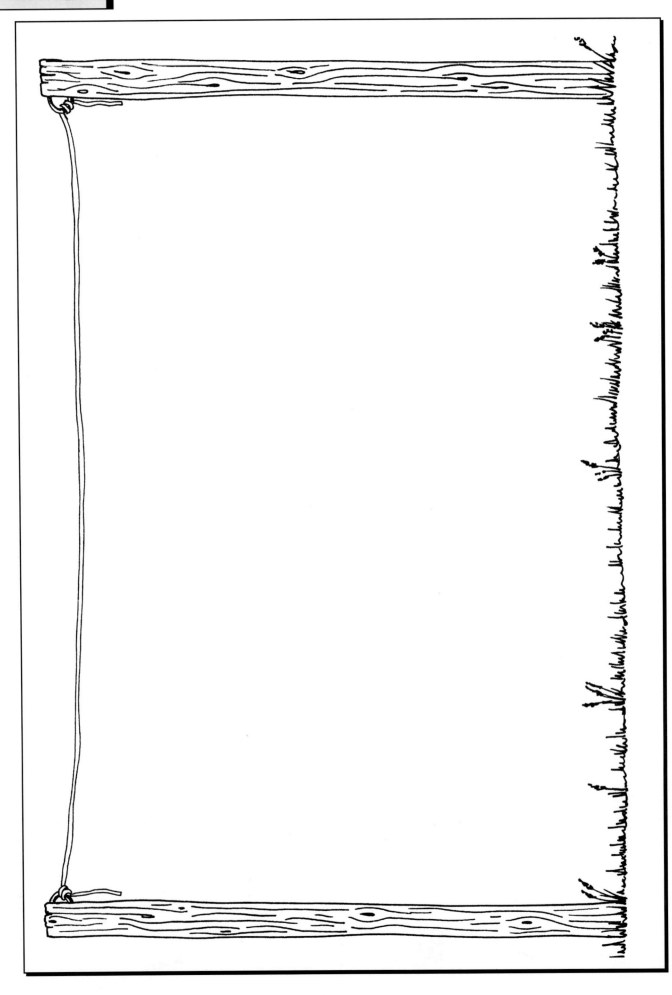

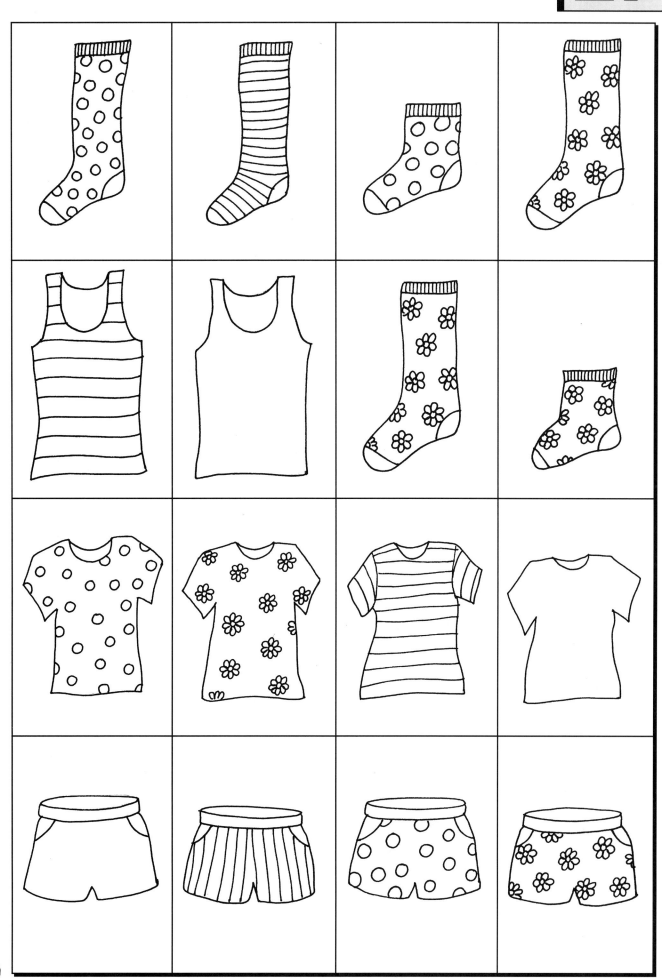

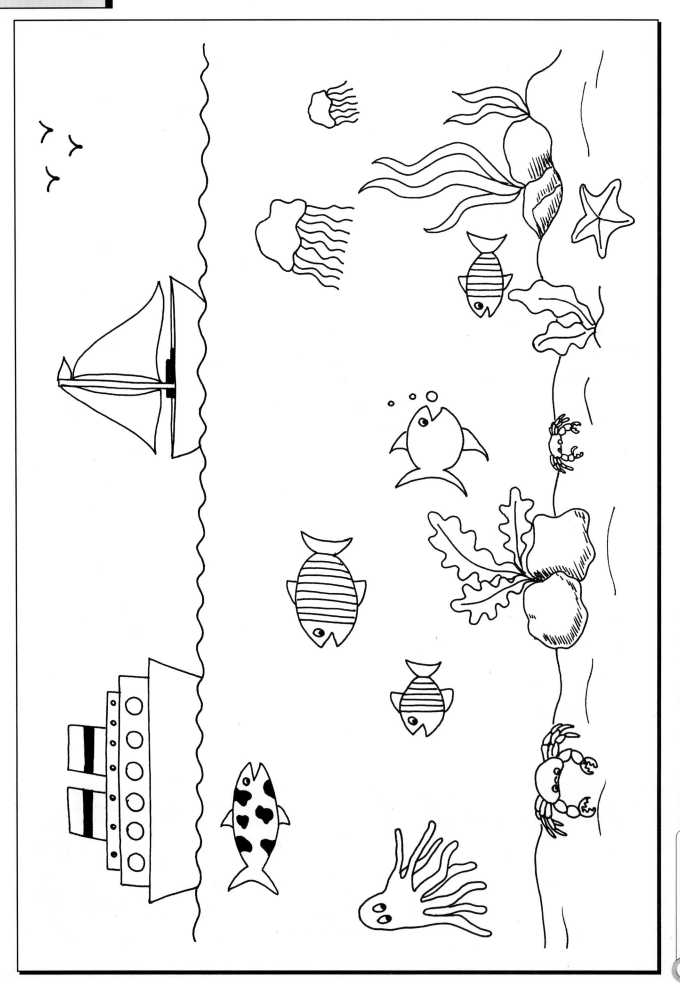

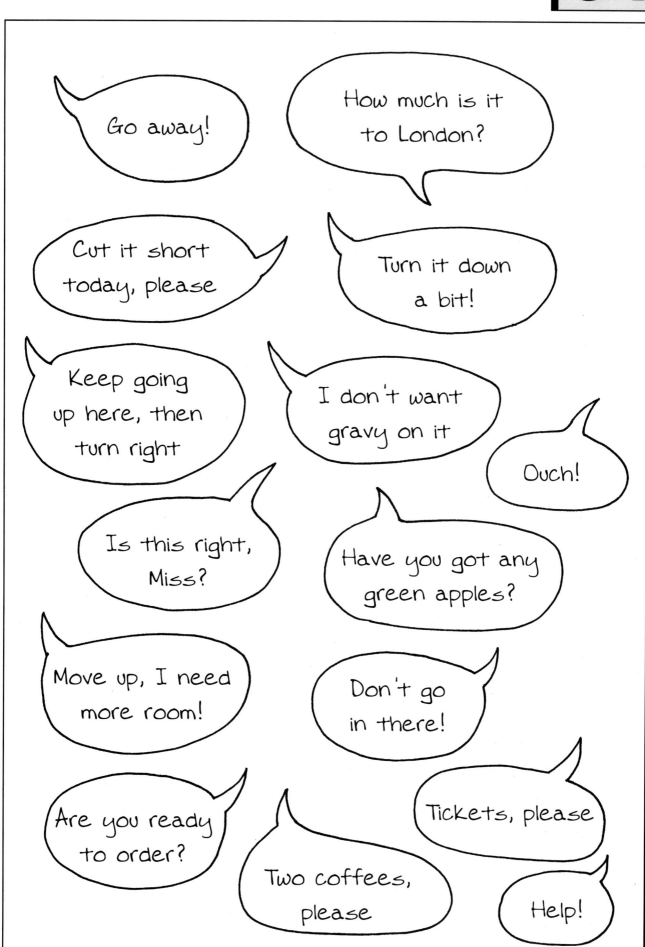

Fires are dangerous	I go to school on Thursdays	Cars can go very fast	Trees lose their leaves in winter
It snows in July	Snails move very fast	I have 30 sisters	People cannot fit in houses
A football floats on water	My house has three bedrooms	I have two brothers	Flowers need water to grow
My hair is bright green	Cornflakes grow on trees	I get up at tea-time	Ice creams can shout at you

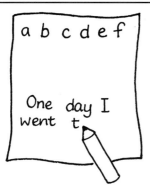

register

1 2 3 4 5 6

$1 + 2 =$

$3 + 1 =$

$5 + 5 =$

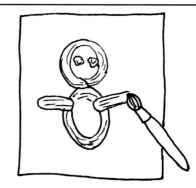

maths

a b c d e f

One day I
went t

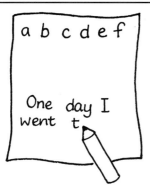

writing

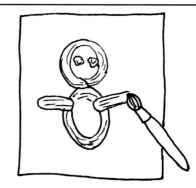

painting

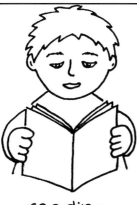

reading

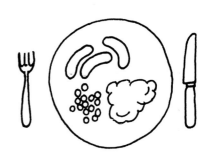

dinner time

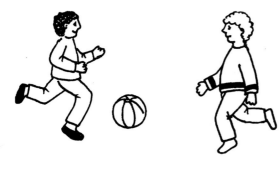

playtime

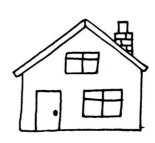

home time

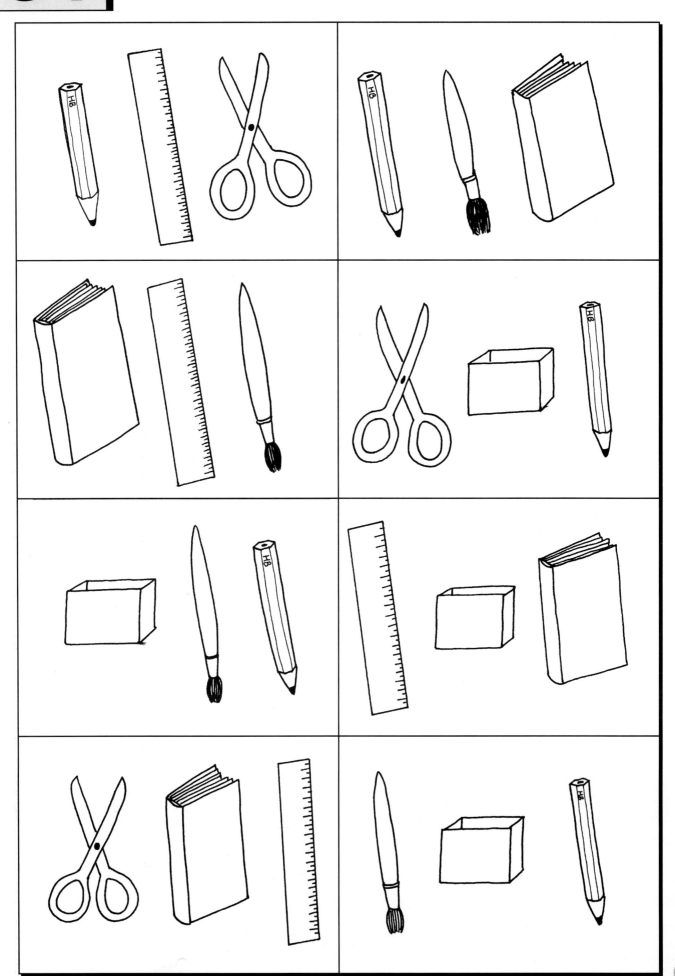

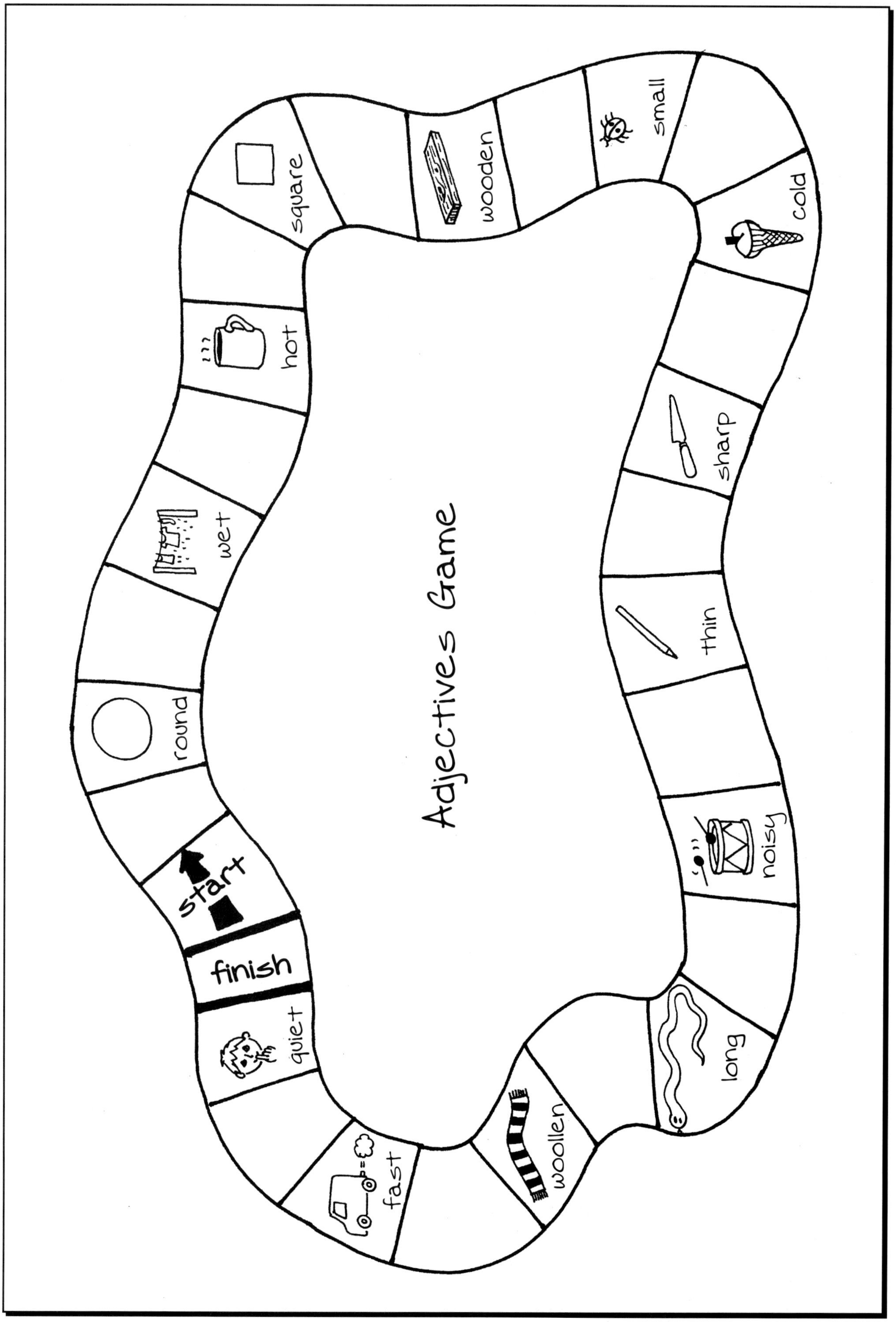

Adjectives Game

small

wooden

square

cold

hot

sharp

wet

thin

round

noisy

start

long

finish

woollen

quiet

fast

36

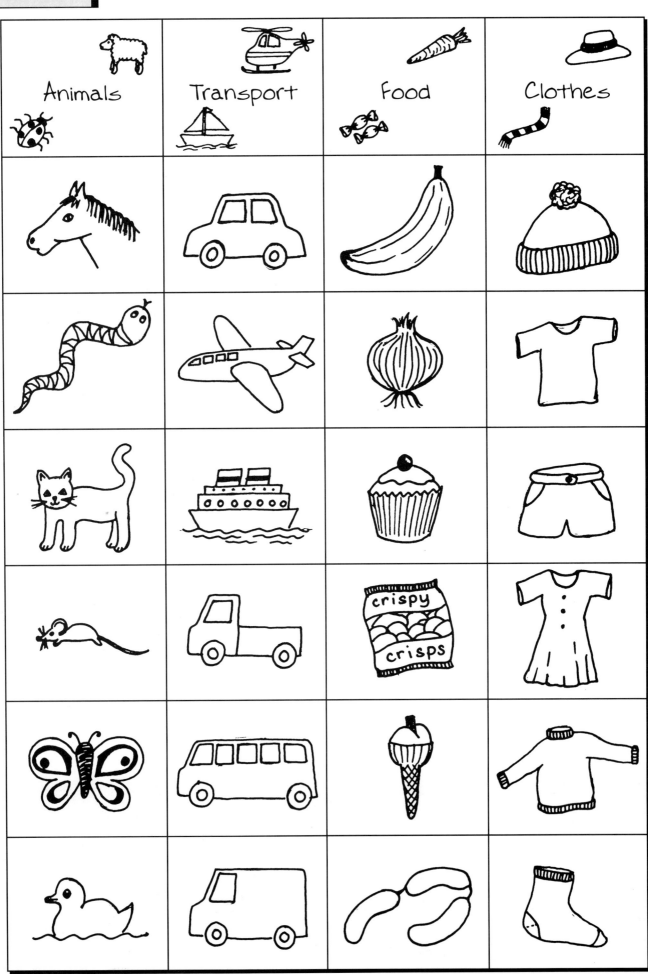

Animals	Transport	Food	Clothes

Summer Clothes	Winter Clothes	Round	Square

Think of ...

start

3 things that can fly

3 animals

2 insects

3 things you can read

4 things you can eat

3 types of transport

4 things you can wear

2 colours

3 toys

3 things made of wood

finish

Odd One Out (1): What are they for?

 pear   sausages   onion   kite

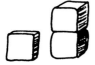 bricks   ball    bed   jigsaw

 vest   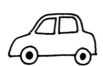 car   shorts   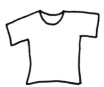 T-shirt

 chair   stool   television   armchair

 cup   plate   glass   mug

 boot   slipper   glove   shoe

Odd One Out (2): Look at the shapes

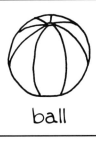 ball

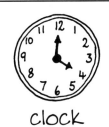 clock

 letter

 face

 mountain

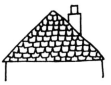 roof

 wizard's hat

 pencil

 egg

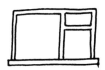 window

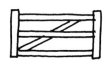 gate

 card

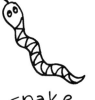 snake

 scarf

 box

 ribbon

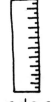 ruler

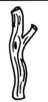 stick

 candle

 kite

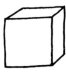 brick

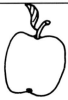 apple

 dice

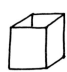 box

Odd One Out (3): Where do you find them?

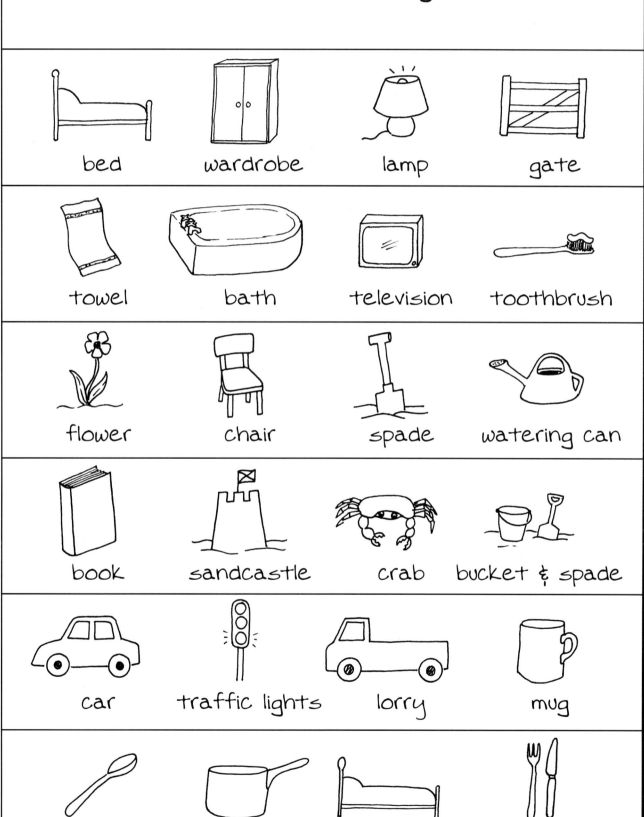

bed	wardrobe	lamp	gate
towel	bath	television	toothbrush
flower	chair	spade	watering can
book	sandcastle	crab	bucket & spade
car	traffic lights	lorry	mug
spoon	pan	bed	knife & fork

Odd One Out (4): Mixed

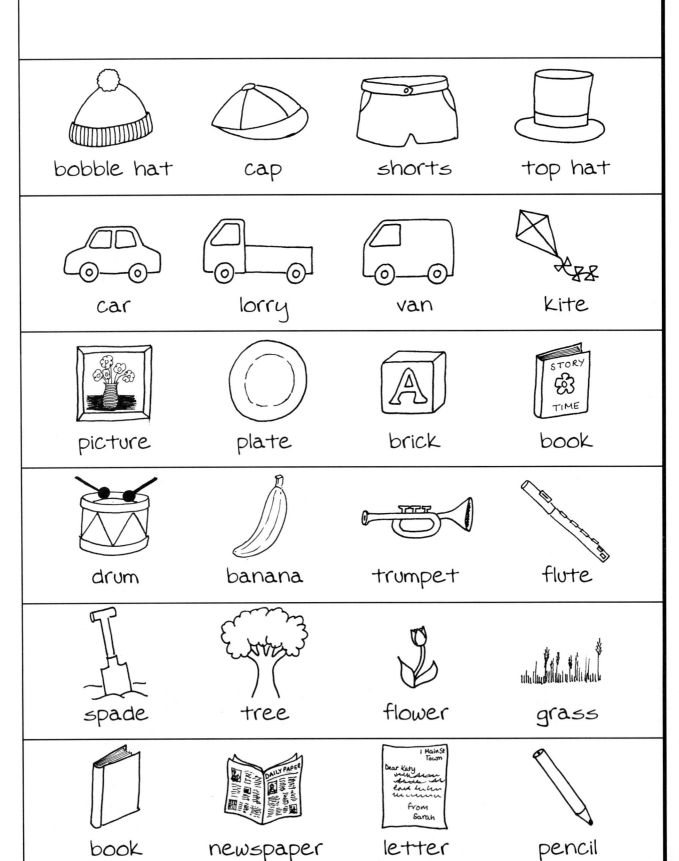

bobble hat	cap	shorts	top hat
car	lorry	van	kite
picture	plate	brick	book
drum	banana	trumpet	flute
spade	tree	flower	grass
book	newspaper	letter	pencil

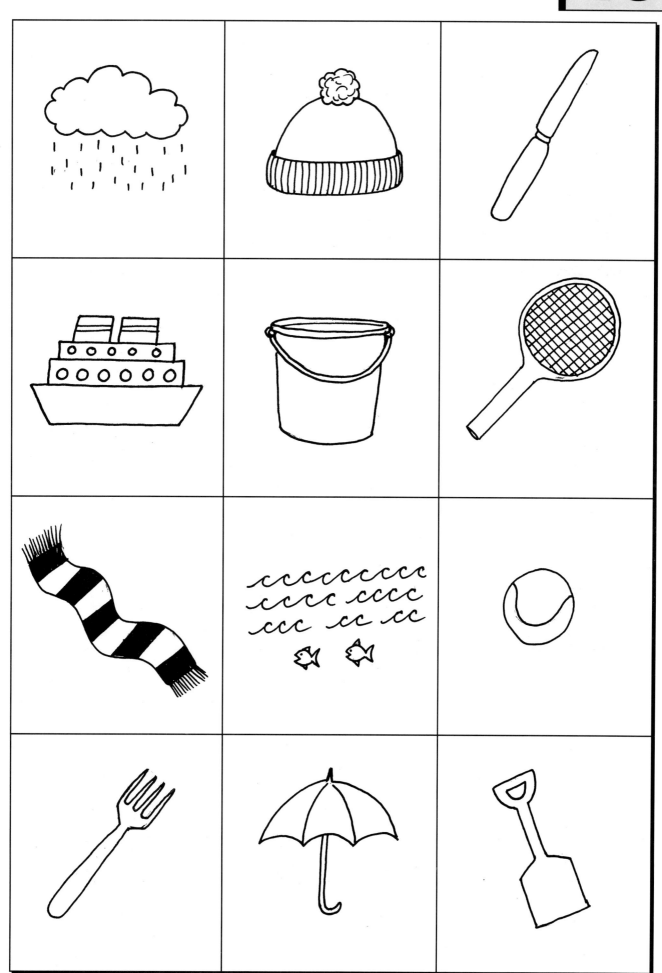

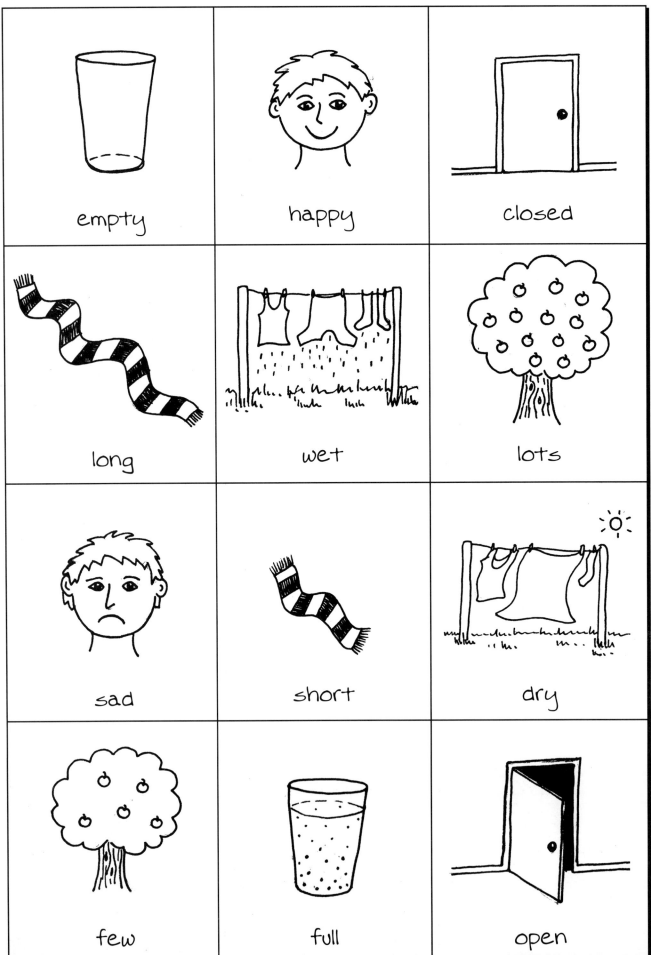

empty	happy	closed
long	wet	lots
sad	short	dry
few	full	open

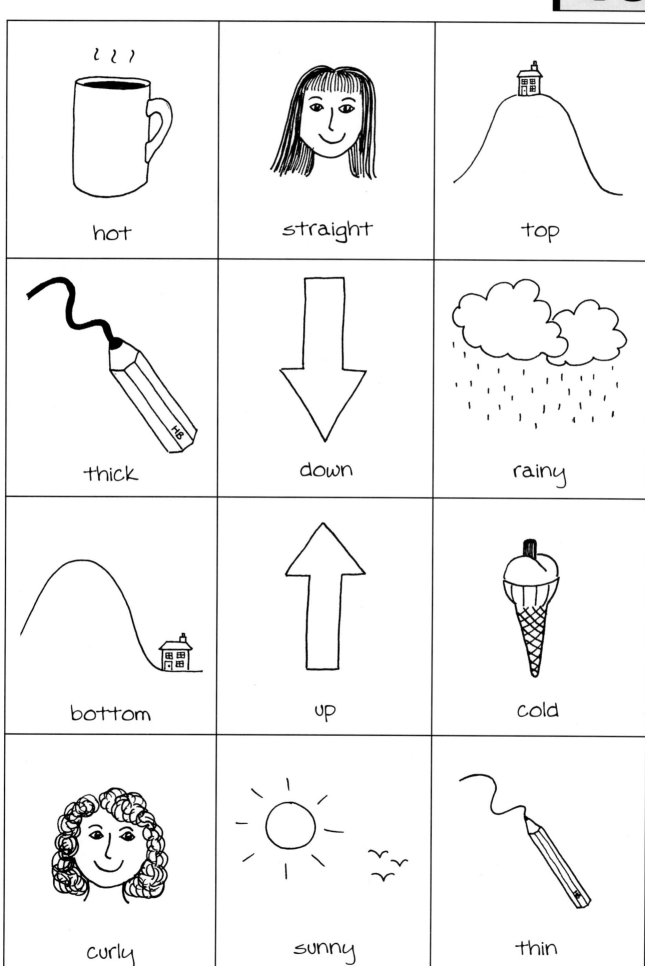

hot	straight	top
thick	down	rainy
bottom	up	cold
curly	sunny	thin

46

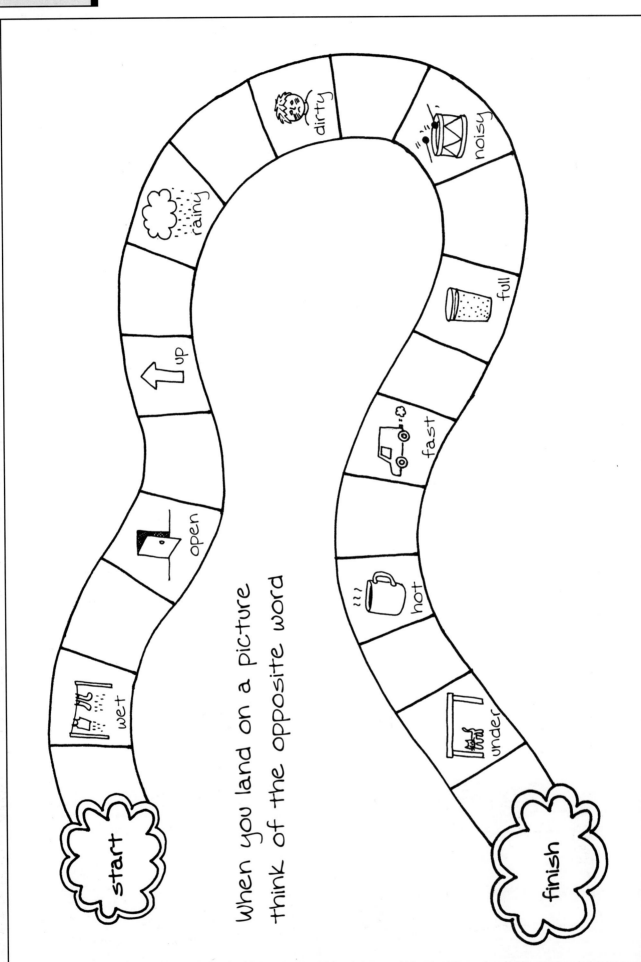

When you land on a picture
think of the opposite word

start

finish

wet

open

up

rainy

dirty

noisy

full

fast

hot

under

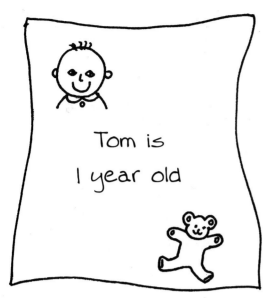

Tom is
1 year old

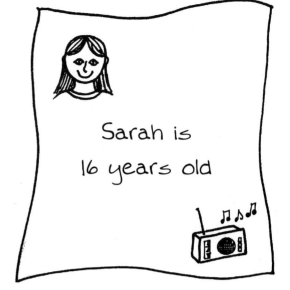

Sarah is
16 years old

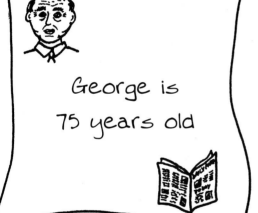

George is
75 years old

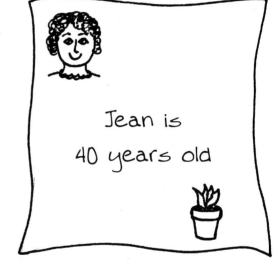

Jean is
40 years old

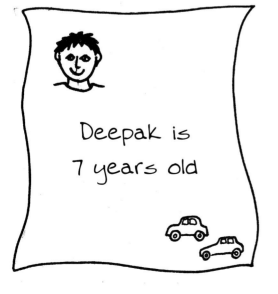

Deepak is
7 years old

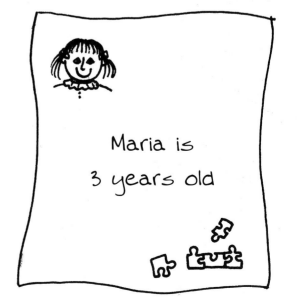

Maria is
3 years old

Mr and Mrs Jones
2 boys and 2 girls,
1 dog.
Mr Jones works
from home.

Mr Symms
Lives alone.
Dislikes gardening.
Likes to be near
shops.

Mr and Mrs McKay
Like the countryside.
Enjoy gardening.

Mrs O'Grady
Retired. Has 2 cats.
Grandchildren come to
stay occasionally.
Likes gardens.
Has a bad back.

Mr and Mrs Gopal
2 teenage children.
Mr Gopal is not at
work, but enjoys DIY.

Mr and Mrs Li
One small baby.
Like to live near
other families.
Dislike DIY.

Mrs Jones has four children and one dog and is always busy.

Mr Symms is 22. He lives alone. Spicy foods are his favourite.

Mr + Mrs McKay have no children. They always take a packed lunch to work. They are vegetarian.

Mrs O'Grady lives alone. She has two cats. She likes to buy treats for her grandchildren.

Mrs Gopal enjoys cooking, especially baking cakes for her family.

Mr + Mrs Li have a small baby. They like to have a cooked breakfast at the weekend.

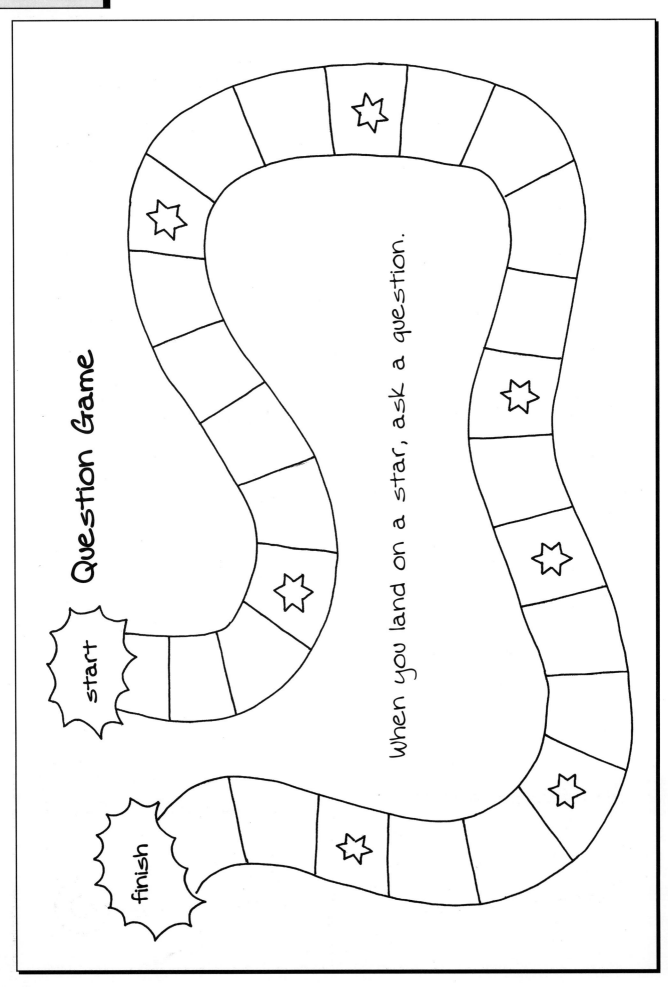

Question Game

start

finish

When you land on a star, ask a question.

51

Who?

Where?

When?

Why?

How?

What?

Are you ...?

Do you...?

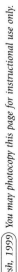

Questionnaire 1

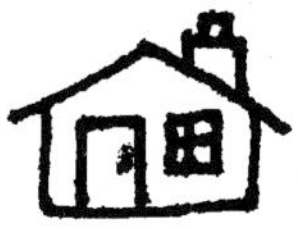

1 Where do you live? _____

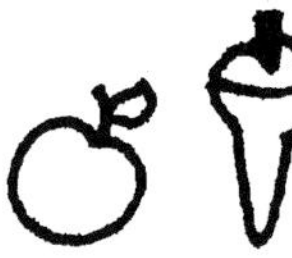

2 What is your favourite food? _____

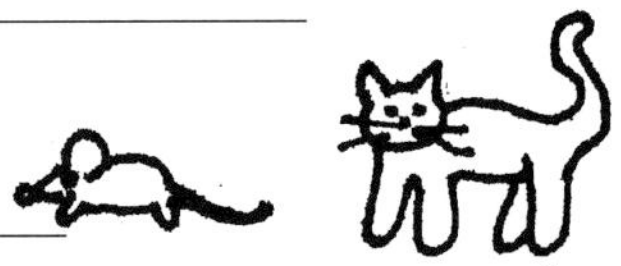

3 Do you have any pets? _____

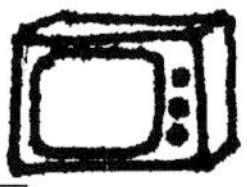

4 What do you like to watch on TV? _____

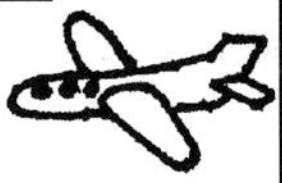

5 Where would you like to go on holiday? _____

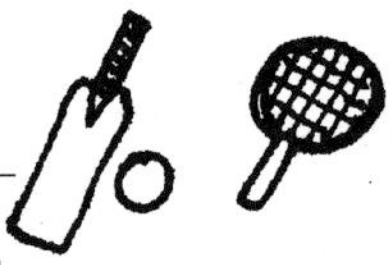

6 What is your favourite sport? _____

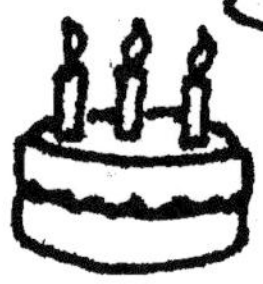

7 When is your birthday? _____

Questionnaire 2

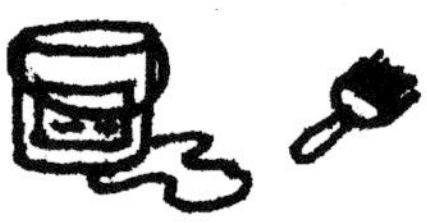

1 What is your favourite colour? _____

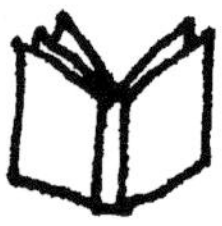

2 What books do you like to read? _____

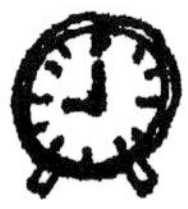

3 What time do you go to bed? _____

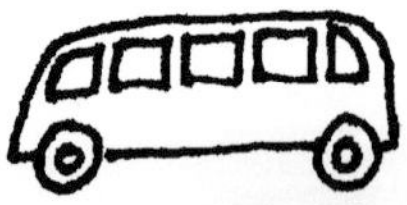

4 How do you get to school? _____

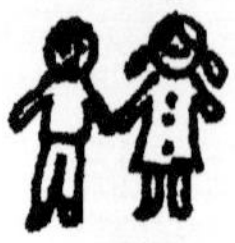

5 Do you have brothers and sisters? _____

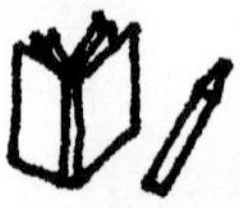

6 What is your favourite school subject? _____

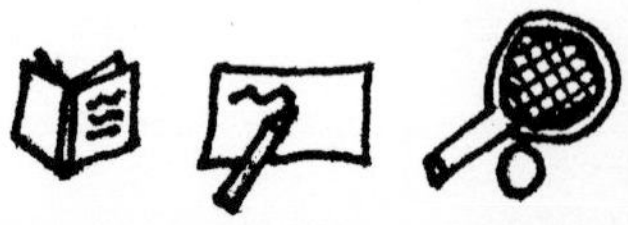

7 What are your hobbies? _____

Can you work it out?

1 I made a cake ... I like chocolate.
   What flavour do you think the cake was?

2 I went to Leeds ... Now I have no money left.
   What did I do in Leeds?

3 I've got a new dress ... It's cotton with no sleeves.
   When will I wear it?

4 I found a book yesterday ... It had pictures of toys
   but no words.   Did I like the book?

5 Someone bought me flowers ... I'm allergic to pollen.
   Did I like the flowers?

6 I put on my thick, coat, scarf and gloves ... Then I
   went outside.   What season was it?

7 I had soup, then fish and chips ... Later I had some
   sponge pudding.   Was I on a diet?

8 "Oh no! I've left the sitting room windows wide open,"
   said Jayne, as she was getting into the car to go
   shopping.   What did Jayne do next?

Can I have a pencil, please?

Give me that pencil!

Move out of the way!

Excuse me, please.

Good morning.

Hiya!

Yuk! I can't stand custard.

I don't really like gravy.

I like your new shoes.

How old are you?

Where do you live?

It's my birthday next week.

Would you like to come to my party?

How many toys have you got?

Your hair looks messy today!

What time is it, please?

Mum or Dad

Aunt or Uncle

Friend

Teacher

Brother
or Sister

Headteacher

Someone at the
bus stop

Neighbour

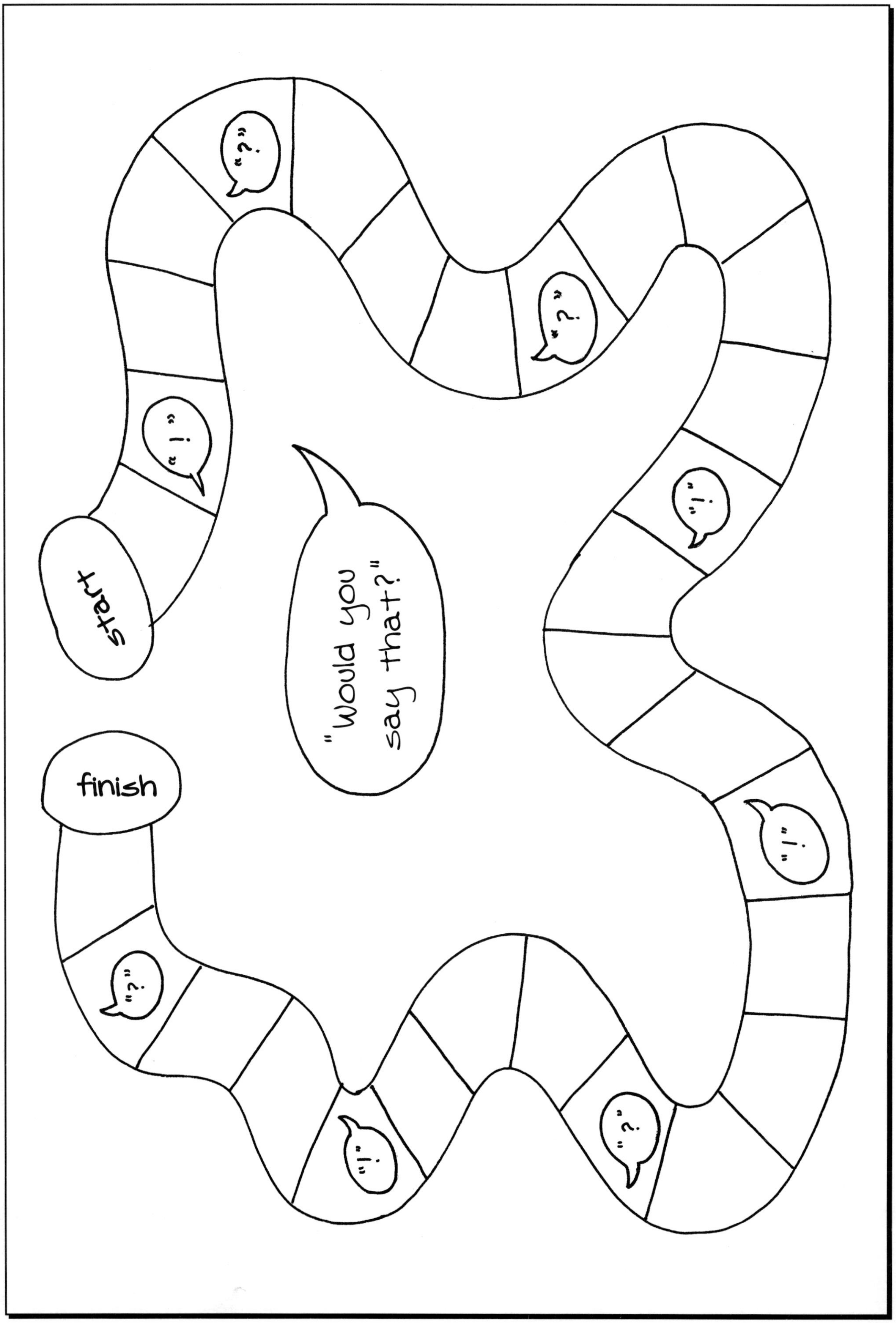

56

start

finish

"Would you say that?"

circular	Mum	fast	hot
approximately	angry	intelligent	cold
fatigued	lovely	next to	sofa
automobile	silly	jumper	bush

58

Shop Assistant

- Should you say anything?
- What might you say?
- How would you say it?

Brother or Sister

- Should you say anything?
- What might you say?
- How would you say it?

Teacher

- Should you say anything?
- What might you say?
- How would you say it?

Some older pupils chatting in a group

- Should you say anything?
- What might you say?
- How would you say it?

Man in a ticket office at the train station

- Should you say anything?
- What might you say?
- How would you say it?

Group of boys playing in the street

- Should you say anything?
- What might you say?
- How would you say it?

Men coming out of a pub

- Should you say anything?
- What might you say?
- How would you say it?

A woman walking down the street or standing at the bus stop

- Should you say anything?
- What might you say?
- How would you say it?